American Dietetic Association Guide to

Gestational Diabetes Mellitus

Alyce M. Thomas, RD, and Yolanda M. Gutierrez, MS, PhD, RD

**American
Dietetic
Association**

Diana Faulhaber, Publisher
Kristen Short, Development Editor
Elizabeth Nishiura, Production Editor

10 9 8 7 6 5 4 3 2

Library of Congress Cataloging-in-Publication Data

Thomas, Alyce M.
  American Dietetic Association guide to gestational diabetes mellitus / Alyce M. Thomas and Yolanda M. Gutierrez.
    p. ; cm. Includes bibliographical references and index.
    ISBN 0-88091-349-5
    1. Diabetes in pregnancy. 2. Diabetes in pregnancy—Diet therapy. I. Gutierrez, Yolanda Monroy. II. American Dietetic Association. III. Title. IV. Title: Guide to gestational diabetes mellitus. [DNLM: 1. Diabetes, Gestational. 2. Nutrition Therapy—Pregnancy.
    WQ 248 T454a 2005]
    RG580.D5T46 2005
    618.3'646—dc22

                                                                          2005010289

REVIEWERS

Molly-Jayne Bangert, RN, CDE
Alamosa, CO

Sharmila Chatterjee, MSc, MS, RD
San Diego, CA

Leona J. Dang-Kilduff, MS, RN, CDE
Palo Alto, CA

Maria Duarte-Gardea, PhD, RD
El Paso, TX

April Eddy, RN, CNS, CDE, APNP
Madison, WI

Tran Hang, MS, RD
Pinellas Park, FL

Laura Hieronymus, MSEd, APRN, BC-ADM, CDE
Lexington, KY

Susan J. Hricko, RN, MSN, CDE, BC-ADM
Sugar Land, TX

Bridget Klawitter, PhD, RD, FADA
Salem, WI

Debi Mann, RN, CDE
St. Louis, MO

Lisa Martin, MA, RD, CDE
Charlotte, NC

Carolé Mensing, MA, RN, CDE
Avon, CT

Emmy Mignano, MS, RD, CDE
Sacramento, CA

Julie M. Moreschi, MS, RD
Lisle, IL

B. Roz Morgan, MPA, RN, CDE
Thousand Oaks, CA

Bethany Newell
Lenexa, KS

Charlotte M. Niznik, MSN, RN, CDE, APN
Chicago, IL

Claire Surr, MEd, APRN, BC-ADM
West Chester, PA

CONTENTS

FOREWORD

Gestational diabetes mellitus, once thought to be a minor complication of pregnancy that was primarily associated with overgrowth of the fetus and that merely needed increased obstetrical surveillance to prevent birth trauma, has come to be recognized as one of the major medical complications of pregnancy. In addition to the concerns about birth trauma, we now know that the metabolic consequences of a hostile intrauterine environment can cause subsequent adult diseases. The literature now supports the relationship between fetal "overnutrition," in the form of hyperglycemia coming from the mother, and the intrauterine development of visceral adiposity, with the consequences of childhood obesity, teenage diabetes, and eventually the full-blown adult cardiovascular metabolic syndrome.

The most common and significant neonatal complication clearly associated with gestational diabetes is neonatal macrosomia: an oversized baby with a birthweight greater than the 90th percentile for gestational age and sex, or a birthweight greater than two standard deviations above the normal mean birth weight. If the fetal macrosomia associated with maternal diabetes mellitus is directly related to maternal glucose concentrations, then strategies to prevent hyperglycemia must be devised to treat the pregnant woman with diabetes. However, not only is the concept controversial that macrosomia is directly related to maternal hyperglycemia, but also the notion that normalizing the maternal glucose could prevent macrosomia is hotly debated.

Some health care professionals believe that an obese woman is at risk for bearing an obese infant independent of the maternal glucose status. However, obese women can only sustain obesity if they are constantly in the fed state. The postprandial glucose concentration of a normal glucose-tolerant woman is higher than her fasting glucose concentration. Thus, an obese woman has a higher mean glucose level than a lean woman, because she is eating most of her waking life. A major controversy in the field of obstetrical nutrition is the safety and efficacy of energy restriction during pregnancy for an obese pregnant woman. The optimal diet for an obese, normoglycemic pregnant woman has not been agreed upon; there is even less consensus on the diet of obese women with gestational diabetes. Thus, if an obese woman with gestational diabetes is fed too much, even though her postprandial glucose concentrations are documented to be normal, she has the additional risk of neonatal macrosomia if her energy intake is not restricted.

In addition, the definition of normoglycemia during pregnancy has not been adequately reported, because of the difficulty of measuring glucose excursions in the home setting. The initial attempts to normalize the 24-hour glucose profile were all done in hospitalized patients. When self-monitoring of blood glucose became available for outpatient surveillance of glucose control, normalization programs could be continued at home. However, the number and timing of the blood glucose determinations have not been adequately studied. In addition, reports that macrosomia occurred despite normoglycemia perpetuated the notion that it is urgent to deliver the infant early, to avoid fetal overgrowth perceived to be unaffected by glycemic control. Perhaps the debate remains because many of the reports that claim that neonatal complications occur despite excellent metabolic control fail to measure postprandial glucose levels. The literature now attests that maternal postprandial glucose concentrations are the most important risk factor in the etiology of macrosomia. The observation that the 1-hour peak postprandial glucose level correlates with the fetal abdominal circumference lends credence to the notion that unless we blunt the peak postprandial response, we shall not be able to impact the macrosomia rate in pregnant women with diabetes. Thus, we must follow protocols of monitoring the postprandial peak glucose concentration and provide optimal meal plans that minimize the peak and yet provide adequate nutrition for the mother and her fetus.

Although normoglycemia is the accepted goal for the management of gestational diabetes, the means to that end remain controversial. Dietary management has been used for the treatment of pregnancies complicated by diabetes since the 19th century; however, a consensus has not been reached as to the optimal diet for the nutrition management of gestational diabetes in lean or obese women. The logical extension to the notion that maternal obesity and hyperglycemia are the major causes of neonatal macrosomia would be to provide an optimal diet as the mainstay of treatment for gestational diabetes. If gestational diabetes is defined as "glucose intolerance," then a diet that minimizes weight gain and provides minimal energy from carbohydrate would be optimal. If we wait for the definitive evidence-based medicine to establish the nutrition therapy for gestational diabetes, we will have lost the opportunity to improve the outcome of pregnancy for a whole generation. There is sufficient science available to provide guidelines and protocols to improve the outcome now.

To provide the best nutrition therapy for women with gestational diabetes, the entire team needs to understand the impact of the disease, to ensure that normoglycemia has been achieved. The dietary principles must not only normalize the blood glucose and maintain the target postprandial glucose concentrations, but they must also provide the necessary vitamins, minerals, and hydration requisite for a pregnant woman. To this end, this book is a magnificent contribution to the field of diabetes and pregnancy. The text has a comprehensive review of all areas of gestational diabetes—pathophysiology, screening and diagnosis, monitoring, and treatment, including the criteria for the initiation of insulin therapy. The book also reviews the optimal diets for gestational diabetes and suggests protocols that have proven to be successful and that result in the birth of healthy infants.

As we wait for the definitive literature to prove that maternal normoglycemia prevents fetal macrosomia and subsequent adult disease, we can follow the wisdom put forth in this book by an incredible team of scientists in the field of the nutrition management of gestational diabetes, Alyce Thomas, RD, and Yolanda M. Gutierrez, MS, PhD, RD. With careful attention to the optimal nutrition of women with gestational diabetes, glucose-mediated macrosomia can be minimized. This book should be used as a resource and considered authoritative for all clinicians who care for women with gestational diabetes.

LOIS JOVANOVIC, MD
Director and Chief Scientific Officer, Sansum Diabetes Research Institute
Clinical Professor of Medicine, University of Southern California
Adjunct Professor of Biomolecular Science and Engineering,
  University of California-Santa Barbara

PREFACE

The importance of nutrition intervention in the treatment and management of gestational diabetes mellitus (GDM) is well established. The *American Dietetic Association Guide to Gestational Diabetes Mellitus* provides a resource for health professionals involved in the care of women who develop diabetes during their pregnancy. This book is intended for dietetics professionals, diabetes educators, physicians, nurses, and other allied health professionals.

The nutrition needs of women with GDM pose a unique challenge to health professionals. Maintaining normoglycemia after the diagnosis of GDM is not the only focus; the provision of adequate energy for normal fetal growth and the promotion of appropriate maternal weight gain are other factors that must be addressed. The goal of this publication is to promote sound nutrition principles in GDM, to achieve optimal outcomes for the woman and her infant. Principles included in this book are not limited to pregnancy but cover the postpartum period as well. The dietary principles learned by women during pregnancy may have a lifelong positive impact on their health and may decrease their risk of developing diabetes in the future.

The topics included in this publication include a historical overview of the management of gestational diabetes in Chapter 1, with a look at the evolution of medical nutrition therapy before the discovery of insulin. Chapter 2 provides a brief discussion of the major physiological changes in energy metabolism and the pathophysiology of GDM.

The criteria for diagnosing GDM are different from those used to diagnose diabetes in nonpregnant individuals. A discussion on screening and diagnosis is included in Chapter 3.

Complications that precede conception or develop during pregnancy can affect the outcome. Chapter 4 highlights maternal and fetal complications associated with GDM. Chapter 5 describes the laboratory tests performed in GDM, with a discussion on method of fetal surveillance.

Medical nutrition therapy is the cornerstone of treatment in the management of GDM. Chapter 6 focuses on this topic, with a brief description of the evidence-based guidelines for

GDM developed by the American Dietetic Association. The chapter also discusses nutrient requirements and the implementation of medical nutrition therapy in GDM.

Chapter 7 explores medications used in the treatment of GDM. This chapter includes a discussion on multivitamin, mineral, and herbal supplement use in pregnancy. Chapter 8 addresses additional concerns that could possibly affect the outcome of pregnancy, including exercise and substance abuse.

Cultural issues that can have an impact on pregnancy are addressed in Chapter 9. The last chapter (Chapter 10) shifts the focus from pregnancy to the postpartum period, with a discussion on the benefits of breastfeeding and the nutritional requirements of the lactating woman who had GDM. The screening criteria for possible postpartum diabetes are also addressed.

The appendixes provide the reader with case studies, forms, and nutrition information that can be adapted to any clinical setting.

It is our hope that this clinical guide will become a valuable source of information to health care professionals who use medical nutrition therapy in the management of GDM.

Alyce R. Thomas, RD
Yolanda M. Gutierrez, MS, PhD, RD

1

Historical Background

Alyce M. Thomas, RD

OBJECTIVES After completing this chapter, you will be able to do the following:

1. Discuss the historical treatment of gestational diabetes mellitus (GDM).
2. Explain how medical nutrition therapy evolved as the scientific community learned more about GDM.
3. Define GDM.

INTRODUCTION

Gestational diabetes mellitus (GDM) is defined as any degree of glucose intolerance with onset or first recognition during pregnancy (1). The definition was proposed at the Second International Workshop-Conference on Gestational Diabetes in 1980 and was subsequently adopted by the American Diabetes Association (2,3). Today, gestational diabetes affects approximately 7% of all pregnant women; 200,000 cases are diagnosed each year (1). The prevalence may range from 1% to 14% of all pregnancies, depending on the population studied and the diagnostic tests used. The incidence in African Americans, Hispanics, American Indians, Asians, and Pacific Islanders is two to four times higher than in non-Hispanic white women (4).

The management of GDM has changed considerably since the 19th century, and its diagnosis and treatment have improved significantly. This chapter examines how the understanding of GDM and treatment modalities have evolved to the standards of practice and guidelines in place today.

EARLY PREINSULIN TREATMENT

One of the earliest recorded cases of GDM occurred in the beginning of the 19th century, when a German woman pregnant with her fifth child began to experience symptoms (polyuria, polydipsia, glycosuria), at 7 months' gestation, that were similar to those of diabetes mellitus. These symptoms had not occurred in her first three pregnancies, but in her fourth pregnancy she had developed polyuria and polydipsia, which ended after delivery. In her fifth pregnancy, the woman was treated with bloodletting and a high-protein diet, and at 36 weeks' gestation, she delivered a 12-pound stillborn baby after very difficult labor. The physician noted an improvement in the woman's condition after delivery, and glucose was no longer detected in her urine. She was discharged with no record of further postpartum care (5).

In the late 19th century, Duncan reviewed 22 cases of diabetes in pregnancy and noted that the fetal death rate was 50%. He observed that diabetes may occur during pregnancy but may be absent at other times; that the infants tended to be enormous; and that the diabetes may end with the termination of the pregnancy but may return sometime afterward (6). In the early 20th century, Joslin observed a number of pregnant women whose symptoms of diabetes disappeared after delivery but often recurred in subsequent pregnancies and, in certain cases, progressed to diabetes (7).

RESEARCH FROM THE 1920s TO 1960s

After the discovery of insulin, maternal survival rates improved, but fetal mortality rates remained high. Although the appearance of glucose in the urine was a common occurrence in pregnancy, it was unclear as to why some women developed diabetes. In 1931, Rowe et al observed a relationship between glycemia and glycosuria during pregnancy (8). The researchers found that glycemic levels were low normal or slightly subnormal throughout pregnancy but returned to normal in the early postpartum period. Like Joslin, they observed that the appearance of glucose in the urine during pregnancy was not uncommon, even in women without diabetes. Richardson and Bitter believed that pregnancy placed a strain on the sugar metabolizing apparatus (9). Their 1932 study involving 247 women was intended to determine why glycosuria occurred in pregnancy and whether this was a serious condition. Eight percent of the women in the study showed a blood glucose curve analogous to that of diabetes mellitus or lowered carbohydrate tolerance. Glycosuria was observed in 42% of the women after delivery, but 50% showed little or no trace of glucose in their urine 12 days postpartum. The cause of the glycosuria in pregnancy could be either high blood glucose levels in the presence of a normal renal threshold similar to that of diabetes mellitus or a lower renal threshold with normal blood glucose levels. Richardson and Bitter suggested that a possible cause of glycosuria was damage to the kidney tubules, which caused the excretion of larger amounts of microscopic sugar crystals (9). A 1946 review article by Eastman found no difference in the treatment modalities of women with diabetes occurring during pregnancy and women with preexisting diabetes (10).

In 1954, Hoet and Lukens observed that pregnancy provoked a disturbance in carbohydrate metabolism, which was evidenced by the hypoglycemic tolerance curve (11). The curve became abnormal around the fourth month of pregnancy but disappeared or diminished from the day of delivery, whether or not glycosuria was present. The fetal mortality rate was in proportion to the increasing severity of the abnormal carbohydrate metabolism. Insulin was used to normalize carbohydrate metabolism, and a reduction in fetal deaths ensued. Correction of the temporary hyperglycemia of pregnancy by insulin could also prevent permanent diabetes later in life.

Diabetes that occurred in pregnancy was often termed "mild" or "transitory" diabetes. In studies published in 1952 and 1960, respectively, Reis et al (12) and Hagbard and Svanborg (13) noted that this form of diabetes was of shorter duration and less severe than preexisting diabetes. In most women, the symptoms disappeared, and oral glucose tolerance test results were normal after delivery. Reis observed that most women with mild diabetes during pregnancy were older and obese (12).

In a 1960 article, Jackson used the term "prediabetes" to indicate the condition in which women produced large babies and tended to develop diabetes mellitus later in life (14). This term had previously been used by Hoet and Lukens in 1954 (11) and by Moss and Mulholland in 1951 (15), to describe women who developed type 2 diabetes after developing transitory diabetes in earlier pregnancies. In studies from the mid-20th century, women with prediabetes had a fetal loss rate of 20% to 67%, and women with prediabetes whose pregnancies ended with live births had a higher rate (20%) of large-for-gestational-age babies (13,16,17).

In 1949, White used the classification "Class A diabetes" to describe diabetes diagnosed for the first time in a pregnant woman with a normal fasting blood sugar and a nondiabetic glucose tolerance test in the early puerperium (18). Dietary restriction was limited, and no insulin therapy was initiated in this class, which had the highest percentage of fetal survival.

O'Sullivan, at Boston General Hospital, was one of the first researchers to use the term "gestational diabetes." In 1961, he categorized gestational diabetes as unsuspected, asymptomatic diabetes that occurred during pregnancy (19). O'Sullivan developed new criteria for the glucose tolerance test in pregnancy. These criteria were used until they were revised by the National Diabetes Data Group (20) in 1980. O'Sullivan proposed that all pregnant women be screened for diabetes with a 1-hour, 50-g glucose test using venous blood (20). If the results were 130 mg/dL or higher, a 3-hour oral glucose tolerance test using the Somogyi-Nelson criteria was given. The patient was instructed to eat 250 g carbohydrate daily for 3 days before the test.

EVOLUTION OF MEDICAL NUTRITION THERAPY FOR GDM

Since the early days of diabetes treatment, medical nutrition therapy has been an essential component in treatment, although various nutrition plans have evolved. In the early 20th century, for example, Naunyn, a physician in Germany, treated diabetic pregnant women with diets that were high in protein and fat (85% of total energy intake) and contained low levels of carbohydrate (21). In severe cases, subjects were treated with starvation diets. There is no indication as to whether the women had preexisting or gestational diabetes.

In 1937, White, of the Joslin Clinic in Boston, treated diabetic pregnant women with a diet that consisted of 30 kcal/kg of body weight, 1 g protein/kg actual body weight, liberal amounts of carbohydrate (180 to 250 g), and the remaining energy intake as fat. White's management protocol included insulin initiation and weekly antepartum visits (22). In 1951, Duncan devised a diet plan similar to White's, but it differed in the protein calculation (the ideal body weight was multiplied by $7/8$ to determine the protein level) and in the energy intake (the ideal body weight in pounds was multiplied by 10, then 100 kcal was added) (23). If edema was present, sodium intake was moderately restricted (no more than 3 g/day); sodium was further reduced if water retention increased. Four to 8 g of ammonium chloride were given daily for 3 days, with a rest period of 2 or 3 days. A quart of milk was added for adequate calcium.

In 1952, Reis et al prescribed a restricted diet to keep hyperglycemia and glycosuria under control (12). Energy intake was based on the woman's nutritional status and activity

TABLE 1.1   Nutrition Management of Gestational Diabetes, 1900 to 1950s

Year	Authors (Reference)	Energy	Carbohydrate	Protein	Fat
1898–1914	Naunyn (21)	Unknown	≤15%	85% (with fat)	
1937	White (22)	30 kcal/kg BW	≥150 g	1 g/kg ABW	Remainder of calories
1951	Duncan (23)	[IBW (lb) × 10] + 100 kcal	180–250 g	IBW × $^7/_8$	Remainder of calories
1951	Moss, Mulholland (15)	30 kcal/kg optimal BW	Added to supply 50 g to fetus	2 g/kg BW	Remainder of calories
1952	Reis et al (12)	25 kcal/kg BW (light work); 30 kcal/kg BW (moderate work)	Unknown	Unknown	Remainder of calories

Abbreviations: ABW, actual body weight; BW, body weight; IBW, ideal body weight.

level: from 25 kcal/kg body weight for light work to 30 kcal/kg for moderate work. In a 1951 article, Moss and Mulholland used 30 kcal/kg of optimal body weight with 2 g/kg body weight of protein for their diet therapy; sufficient carbohydrate was added to supply 50 g/day to the fetus and an adequate amount for the woman, with the remainder as fat (15). Sodium was restricted, and the woman was advised to gain no more than 20 lb.

For a summary of nutrition management strategies used by researchers in the early 19th and mid-20th centuries, see Table 1.1 (12,15,21–23). Medical nutrition therapy plans implemented today can be found in Chapter 6.

RESEARCH FROM THE 1960s TO THE 1980s

Researchers from the 1960s to the 1980s associated several maternal and fetal factors, including obesity, age, and macrosomia, with gestational diabetes. Weight loss was recommended for obese pregnant women, with energy intake restricted to 20 kcal/kg ideal body weight. In the mid-1970s, Pedersen treated obese pregnant women with a 1,200-kcal diet and metformin (24). Insulin was initiated if glycemic levels remained elevated. Macrosomia was observed in the infants of women with transient diabetes, with birth weights of more than 5,000 g. The mothers of these infants with macrosomia were often obese (14,25). Infants were often delivered early (35 to 37 weeks' gestation), to decrease the risk of fetal death (11). As early as 5 years after delivery, the incidence of type 2 diabetes was observed to be higher in women with gestational diabetes than in women without gestational diabetes (25).

From the 1940s through the 1960s, weight gain had been routinely restricted during pregnancy, including in women with diabetes, to decrease the risk of hypertension. It was considered normal practice for women to gain less than 20 lb. This regimen continued until the release of the 1970 National Research Council's report *Maternal Nutrition and the Course of Pregnancy,* which showed evidence that restricting maternal weight gain could have long-term adverse consequences for the growth and development of the fetus (26). The weight gain restriction was eased to 22 to 30 lb for women without diabetes, but this recommendation did not apply to women with gestational or preexisting diabetes. For these women, to avoid the risks associated with diabetes and pregnancy, the recommendation was to gain minimal amounts of weight (<15 lb) (27).

However, research never proved that moderate weight gain by a pregnant woman with any type of diabetes had an adverse effect on the fetus. In 1979, the weight restrictions for pregnant women with diabetes were relaxed to those recommended for pregnant women without diabetes (28). Medical nutrition therapy was modified to reflect the American Diabetes Association's recommendations for nonpregnant women with diabetes, which suggested moderate amounts of complex carbohydrates and no refined sugars. The intake of cholesterol and saturated fats was also limited (28).

DEVELOPMENT OF GDM RECOMMENDATIONS

The definition of GDM—glucose intolerance recognized during pregnancy—was initially established during the First International Conference-Workshop on Gestational Diabetes Mellitus (29). The recommendations included universal screening for all women between the 24th and 28th weeks of pregnancy. The diagnosis of GDM was in accordance with the O'Sullivan criteria of two or more values from the 3-hour oral glucose tolerance test exceeding the following plasma glucose values (29,30):

- Fasting: 105 mg/dL
- 1-hour: 190 mg/dL
- 2-hour: 165 mg/dL
- 3-hour: 145 mg/dL

As in the earlier days of gestational diabetes treatment, medical nutrition therapy was considered an essential component of the treatment modality. Insulin was initiated when medical nutrition therapy failed to maintain a fasting plasma glucose value of less than 105 mg/dL and a 2-hour postprandial value of less than 120 mg/dL.

At the Second International Workshop-Conference on Gestational Diabetes in 1984, the definition of GDM was expanded to include whether or not insulin was used or whether the condition persisted after pregnancy. This definition was subsequently adopted by the American Diabetes Association (2,3). The Second International Workshop-Conference on Gestational Diabetes recommended the use of the 50-g glucose load in screening for glucose intolerance (2). The 100-g oral glucose tolerance test using O'Sullivan's criteria was used if the glucose load was 140 mg/dL or higher. The 75-g oral glucose tolerance test was used to diagnose postpartum diabetes. If insulin was initiated, self-monitoring of blood glucose levels was recommended.

The summary of the Third International Workshop-Conference (published in 1991) emphasized fetal macrosomia as a risk factor for GDM (31). Other factors that were reported to predispose women to developing GDM included maternal age, obesity, ethnicity, gestational age, past obstetrical history, and family history of diabetes (31). The National Diabetes Data Group's criteria were again used as the standard for screening and diagnosing for GDM.

SUMMARY

GDM is defined as glucose intolerance with onset or first recognition during pregnancy. Although the treatment of GDM has changed since the discovery of insulin, certain morbidities, such as fetal macrosomia, are more prevalent in women with GDM than in healthy women.

The management of diabetes during pregnancy has changed since the early 19th century. Early medical nutrition therapy consisted of various regimens, ranging from starvation diets to high-protein/high-fat diets to low-calorie diets. Three international conferences on GDM have formalized the definition and established screening and diagnosis criteria.

REFERENCES

1. American Diabetes Association. Position statement. Gestational diabetes mellitus. *Diabetes Care.* 2004;27(Suppl 1):S88–S90.

2. Freinkel N. Summary and recommendations of the Second International Workshop-Conference on Gestational Diabetes. *Diabetes.* 1985;34(Suppl. 2):S123–S126.

3. Coustan DR, Carpenter MW. The diagnosis of gestational diabetes. *Diabetes Care.* 1998;21(Suppl 2):B5–B8.

4. Centers for Disease Control and Prevention. Diabetes and women's health across the life stages: a public health perspective. Available at: http://www.cdc.gov/diabetes/pubs/pdf/women.pdf. Accessed December 7, 2004.

5. Hadden DR. A historical perspective on gestational diabetes. *Diabetes Care.* 1998;21(Suppl 2):B3–B4.

6. Duncan JM. On puerperal diabetes. *Trans London Obstet Soc.* 1882;24:256–285.

7. Joslin EP. Pregnancy and diabetes. *Boston Med Surg J.* 1915;173:841–849.

8. Rowe AW, Gallivan DE, Matthews H. The metabolism of pregnancy: the carbohydrate metabolism. *Am J Physiol.* 1931;96:94–100.

9. Richardson R, Bitter RS. Glycosuria in pregnancy. *Am J Obstet Gynecol.* 1932;24:362–369.

10. Eastman NJ. Diabetes mellitus and pregnancy: a review. *Obstet Gynecol Surv.* 1946;1:3–31.

11. Hoet JP, Lukens FD. Carbohydrate metabolism during pregnancy. *Diabetes.* 1954;3:1–12.

12. Reis RA, DeCosta EJ, Allweiss MD. *Diabetes and Pregnancy.* Springfield, Ill: Charles C. Thomas; 1952.

13. Hagbard L, Svanborg A. Prognosis of diabetes mellitus with onset during pregnancy: a clinical study of seventy-one cases. *Diabetes.* 1960;9:296–302.

14. Jackson WP. Present status of prediabetes. *Diabetes.* 1960;9:373–378.

15. Moss JM, Mulholland HB. Diabetes and pregnancy: with special reference to the prediabetic state. *Ann Intern Med.* 1951;34:678–691.

16. Miller HC. The effect of diabetic and prediabetic pregnancies on the fetus and newborn infant. *J Pediatr.* 1946;29:455–461.

17. Wilkerson HL. Pregnancy and the prediabetic state. *Ann N Y Acad Sci.* 1959;82:219–228.

18. White P. Pregnancy complicating diabetes. *Am J Med.* 1949;7:609–616.

19. O'Sullivan JB. Gestational diabetes: unsuspected, asymptomatic diabetes in pregnancy. *N Engl J Med.* 1961;264:1082–1085.

20. National Diabetes Data Group. Classification and diagnosis of diabetes mellitus and other categories of glucose intolerance. *Diabetes.* 1979;28:1039–1057.

21. Ney D, Hollingsworth DR. Nutritional management of pregnancy complicated by diabetes: historical perspective. *Diabetes Care.* 1981;4:647–655.

22. White P. Diabetes complicating pregnancy. *Am J Obstet Gynecol.* 1937;33:380–385.

23. Duncan GG. *Diabetes Mellitus: Principles & Treatment.* Philadelphia, Pa: WB Saunders; 1951.

24. Pedersen J. *The Pregnant Diabetic and Her Newborn.* 2nd ed. Baltimore, Md: Williams and Wilkins; 1977.

25. O'Sullivan JB, Gellis SS, Tenney BO. Gestational blood glucose levels in normal and potentially diabetic women related to the birth weight of their infants. *Diabetes.* 1966;15:466–470.

26. Committee on Maternal Nutrition/Food and Nutrition Board. *Maternal Nutrition and the Course of Pregnancy.* Washington, DC: National Research Council; 1970.

27. White P. Pregnancy in diabetes. In: Marble A, White P, Bradley R, Krall LP, eds. *Joslin's Diabetes Mellitus.* 11th ed. Philadelphia, Pa: Lea and Febiger; 1971.

28. American Diabetes Association and American Dietetic Association. Principles of nutrition and dietary recommendations for patients with diabetes mellitus. *Diabetes Care.* 1979;2:520–523.

29. American Diabetes Association. Summary and recommendations of the First International Conference-Workshop on Gestational Diabetes Mellitus. *Diabetes Care.* 1980;3:499–501.

30. O'Sullivan JB, Mahan CM. Criteria for the oral glucose tolerance test in pregnancy. *Diabetes.* 1964;13:278–285.

31. Metzger BE. Summary and recommendations of the Third International Workshop-Conference on Gestational Diabetes Mellitus. *Diabetes.* 1991;40(Suppl 2):S197–S201.

Pathophysiology of Gestational Diabetes Mellitus

Alyce M. Thomas, RD

Alyce M. Thomas, RD

OBJECTIVES   After completing this chapter, you will be able to do the following:

1. Describe the major physiological changes in glucose, amino acids, and lipid metabolism in normal pregnancy.
2. Explain the role of insulin and placental hormones in glucose homeostasis.
3. Discuss the effect of gestational diabetes mellitus (GDM) on maternal nutrient metabolism and insulin secretion.
4. Describe the effect of GDM on the fetus.

EFFECTS OF A NORMAL PREGNANCY ON MATERNAL PHYSIOLOGY

During pregnancy, several physiological alterations occur to meet both maternal and fetal energy and nutritional demands. These alterations affect glucose, amino acid, and lipid metabolism, as well as insulin secretion. Table 2.1 (1–3) illustrates the laboratory value differences between nonpregnant women and women with normal pregnancies.

Energy Demands

In the first trimester, elevation of the hormones human placental lactogen (hPL) and cortisol decreases maternal glucose levels (4,5). An increase in serum estrogen and progesterone levels stimulates the production and secretion of additional insulin while increasing insulin sensitivity (5). The result is a decrease in maternal fasting and postprandial glucose levels in the first 12 weeks of gestation (6). Fasting glucose levels in women with normal pregnancies are 10% to 20% lower than in nonpregnant women (7). The lower levels protect the fetus from receiving excessive glucose during the critical period of organogenesis.

TABLE 2.1 Laboratory Values in Nonpregnant Women and Women With Normal Pregnancies

Test	Reference Range* Nonpregnant	Pregnant
Hematology		
Red blood cell count, $\times 10^{12}$/L	4.2–5.4	3.21–4.89
Hemoglobin, g/dL	12.0–16.0	10.0–14.0
Hematocrit, %	38.0–47.0	29.5–41.2
MCV, fL	81.0–99.0	82.4–100.5
MCH, pg	26.0–32.0	27.0–34.8
MCHC, %	32.0–36.0	31.9–35.6
WBC, $\times 10^9$/L	5.0–10.0	3.9–12.9
Lymphocytes, $\times 10^9$/L	1.0–4.0	0.4–1.8
Monocytes, $\times 10^9$/L	0.1–0.7	0.0–0.9
Neutrophils, $\times 10^9$/L	2.5–8.0	2.82–10.18
Platelet count, $\times 10^9$/L	150–400	1.21–3.73
Mean platelet volume, fL	7.4–10.4	6.4–11.6
Chemistry		
Albumin, g/dL	3.5–5.0	2.8–4.3
Alkaline phosphatase, IU/L	31–97	22–267
Bilirubin (total), mg/dL	0.1–1.0	0.0–4.2
BUN, mg/dL	6–19	7–8
Calcium (total), mg/dL	8.4–10.5	7.5–9.4
Cholesterol (total), mg/dL	<200	140–250
Creatinine (serum), mg/dL	0.5–1.1	0.6–1.2
Glucose, mg/dL	70–105	<140
Iron (total), mcg/dL	60–160	50–132
Iron (TIBC), mcg/dL	250–460	265–411
Iron (transferrin), mg/dL	250–380	200–400
Magnesium, mEq/dL	1.3–2.1	1.8–3.0
Phosphorus, mg/dL	3.0–4.5	2.5–5.0
Potassium, mEq/dL	3.5–5.0	3.4–4.9
Protein (total), g/dL	6.0–8.3	5.2–7.2
Sodium (serum), mEq/dL	136–145	31–141
Uric acid (serum), mg/dL	2.4–6.0	2.6–6.0
Urinalysis		
Blood[†]	Negative	
Color[†]	Yellow to amber	
Glucose[†]	Negative	
Ketones[†]	Negative	
pH[†]	4.5–8.0	
Protein[†]	Negative	
Specific gravity[†]	1.015–1.025	
Turbidity[†]	Clear to slightly hazy	
A1C[†], %	2–5 (nondiabetes)	
	<6 (good diabetes control)	
	6–8 (fair diabetes control)	
	>8 (poor diabetes control)	

TABLE 2.1   (continued)

Test	Reference Range*	
	Nonpregnant	Pregnant
Lipid profile—risk factors		
Total cholesterol[†], mg/dL	<200 (desirable)	
	200–239 (borderline-high)	
	≥240 (high)	
HDL cholesterol[†], mg/dL	>60 (optimal)	
	40–59 (borderline-high)	
	<40 (high)	
LDL cholesterol[†], mg/dL	<100 (optimal)	
	100–129 (near optimal)	
	130–159 (borderline-high)	
	160–189 (high)	
	≥190 (very high)	
Triglycerides[†], mg/dL	<150 (optimal)	
	150–199 (borderline-high)	
	200–499 (high)	
	≥500 (very high)	

Abbreviations: BUN, blood urea nitrogen; HDL, high-density lipoprotein; LDL, low-density lipoprotein; MCH, mean corpuscular hemoglobin; MCHC, mean corpuscular hemoglobin concentration; MCV, mean corpuscular volume; TIBC, total iron-binding capacity; WBC, white blood cells.

*Reference values may differ depending on the laboratory.

[†]No reference value is given for pregnancy.

Source: Data are from references 1 through 3.

As glycemic levels rise after eating, the pancreas secretes additional insulin, which returns glucose levels to normal relatively quickly and ensures an adequate supply to the fetus (4). This constant need for glucose by the fetus tends to cause maternal hypoglycemia between meals and during the night (5). The mother's body is able to compensate for this drain on her glycemic levels by an enhanced capacity for nutrient storage during feeding (8). Insulin is responsible for storing the excess maternal calories to lipid and tissue sites for later use.

The placenta regulates maternal and fetal transfer of nutrients (Figure 2.1) (9). Glucose is transported to the fetus through the placenta via facilitated diffusion (8). Fetal glucose concentrations are 10 to 20 mg/dL lower than maternal concentration (7). The placenta contains high concentrations of insulin-dependent glucose transport molecules. These glucose transporters, also called GLUT transporters, assist in the transport of glucose across the placenta (8,10,11). An alteration in the rate of GLUT transporters will result in a change in the circulating glucose concentration. Higher maternal glycemic levels will increase the amount of glucose transported to the fetus.

In the second trimester, as the levels of estrogen, progesterone, and the placental hormones (hPL, prolactin, and cortisol) rise, there is an increase in insulin resistance, a decrease in insulin sensitivity, and higher fasting and postprandial blood glucose levels in the pregnant woman (4,5,12–16). Human placental lactogen is a main contributor to reduced insulin sensitivity and impaired glucose tolerance (5). The increased secretion of hPL also in-

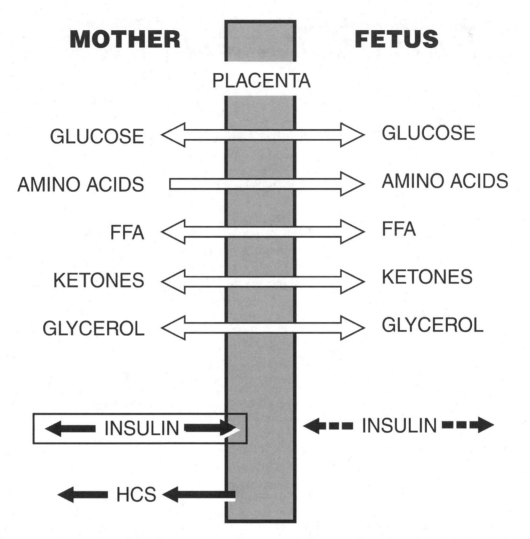

FIGURE 2.1. Placental permeability and the relationship between maternal and fetal fuels. FFA = free fatty acids; HCS = human chorionic somatomammotropin. Reprinted from Frienkel N. Banting Lecture 1980: Of pregnancy and progeny. *Diabetes.* 1980;29:1028–1035. Copyright © 1980 American Diabetes Association. Reprinted with permission from the American Diabetes Association.

hibits the uptake of glucose in peripheral tissues and stimulates fetal pancreatic insulin secretion. Elevated concentration of prolactin blunts insulin action. The rise in maternal cortisol levels increases the hepatic production of glucose (17). As fetal nutrient demands increase, the liver is stimulated to mobilize maternal glucose stores and to increase the concentration of circulating glucose. An increase in insulin resistance places a greater demand on the pancreatic beta cells to secrete additional levels of insulin (7). Maternal insulin resistance continues into the third trimester, resulting in an increase in insulin production that can triple that of nonpregnancy levels to maintain normoglycemia (4).

Protein Needs and Lipid Responses

Protein is essential for fetal and placental growth and development. Amino acids are transferred across the placenta by active transport (18). The plasma levels of amino acids are lower in pregnant women than in nonpregnant women. This is caused by the action of progesterone to increase the hepatic utilization of amino acids, which results in decreased plasma levels (7). Cortisol, prolactin, and hPL also act to ensure that the fetus receives a continuous supply of amino acids (7). As a result of the placental transport, fetal amino acid levels are higher than maternal levels (5,7).

Pregnancy is associated with increased levels of triglycerides, low-density lipoproteins (LDL), high-density lipoproteins (HDL), and total cholesterol (18). During the first half of pregnancy, fat is deposited in the maternal adipose tissues (7). These fat stores are later mobilized, increasing the production of plasma free fatty acids and ketones. In a normal pregnancy, the rise in free fatty acids in pregnancy affects insulin action by causing insulin resistance (19). Free fatty acids may influence the hepatic production of glucose, which results in increased insulin resistance and decreased insulin sensitivity. The pregnant woman uses lipids for energy metabolism, whereas the fetus depends on glucose as its primary fuel source. This may save the fetus during any period of starvation in the pregnant woman. Conversely, if a maternal starvation state exists, the fetus will use ketones transported across the placenta as an energy source. Free fatty acids have been associated with altered fetal growth. It is possible that higher levels of free fatty acids may predispose the fetus to macrosomia (20).

Multiple Gestations

Twin and higher multiple gestations are associated with several adverse effects, including preterm labor, preterm delivery, placenta previa, and premature rupture of the membranes and preeclampsia (21–23). In multiple gestations, placental lactogen levels are higher and placental size is greater. For these reasons, one would expect a higher incidence of GDM than in singleton pregnancies. Studies have shown, however, that no increased risk of GDM was found in multiple gestations (24–30).

EFFECTS OF GDM ON MATERNAL PHYSIOLOGY

GDM is pathophysiologically similar to type 2 diabetes, in that abnormalities in islet cell function or peripheral insulin resistance at the receptor level are thought to decrease insulin secretory response and insulin sensitivity (4,5,11). The inability of the pancreatic beta cell to increase insulin secretion in response to the increased insulin needs during pregnancy possibly results in higher levels of circulating glucose in the bloodstream (18).

There is a general delay in the insulin response to an alteration in glucose metabolism and a more pronounced insulin insensitivity (5,11,12). Insulin-antagonist hormones, particularly hPL, contribute to insulin resistance and a rise in glycemic levels (5).

PREEXISTING FACTORS

Preexisting maternal factors, such as obesity, also affect insulin secretion and resistance. An obese woman with GDM, similar to the nonpregnant woman with type 2 diabetes, may secrete higher levels of insulin than her normal-weight or lean counterpart (7). Obese women are more likely to experience impairment in insulin sensitivity resulting from the ineffective production of hepatic glucose (11). The decrease in insulin sensitivity, possibly caused by the destruction or impaired function of the beta cells, can continue into the postpartum period. This could explain the higher incidence of impaired glucose tolerance or type 2 diabetes in women with previous GDM (31).

Another factor in decreased insulin sensitivity in GDM is maternal weight gain. Insulin receptors are reduced by increased secretion of hPL. As the body attempts to maintain normoglycemia, excessive insulin is released, and the woman experiences increased hunger (5). The increased insulin secretion triggered by elevated hormonal levels results in excess energy intake and subsequent higher-than-recommended weight gain (5). Free amino acids stimulate maternal pancreatic beta cell replication and insulin synthesis (7). Kalkhoff found higher amino acid concentrations in women with GDM than in healthy pregnant women (32). The infant birth weight was significantly correlated with maternal plasma amino acid levels. Levels of maternal free fatty acids tend to be higher in women with GDM than in those without GDM, possibly stimulating excessive fetal growth (20).

EFFECTS OF GDM ON FETAL PHYSIOLOGY

The effect of GDM is not limited to the woman. Fetal physiology is also affected when maternal glycemic levels are elevated. As discussed earlier in this chapter, glucose is the primary fuel source used by the fetus, and it crosses the placenta by facilitated diffusion (10,32). Amino acids, necessary for fetal muscle development, are used in smaller amounts (7). An elevation in the maternal blood glucose will result in a subsequent increase in fetal glucose diffusion. The fetus consistently exposed to higher levels of maternal circulating glucose will experience an increase in fetal insulin production (32,33). Maternal insulin does not cross the placental barrier unless it is bound to IgG antibodies. Insulin acts as a fetal growth hormone, and excessive amounts of insulin (hyperinsulinemia) in response to continual excessive glucose can lead to beta cell hyperplasia and macrosomia. Pedersen hypothesized that maternal hyperglycemia induces fetal hyperglycemia leading to fetal hyperinsulinemia and macrosomia (34). Although large, the infant's organs are not necessarily mature.

The production of insulin in the fetal pancreas begins in the first trimester, at approximately 11 or 12 weeks' gestation (7). It is excreted in the fetal urine and is found in amniotic fluid by the 12th week of pregnancy (7). As the pregnancy advances, the amniotic insulin level increases in response to the fetal secretion of insulin. Excessive or insufficient amniotic fluid insulin levels are associated with fetal morbidity or mortality (7,8). Elevated amniotic fluid insulin levels were correlated with macrosomia (5). Intrauterine growth retardation, preeclampsia, congenital anomalies, and fetal death are associated with abnormally low amniotic fluid insulin levels (7,8).

Small-for-gestational-age fetuses and intrauterine growth retardation are relatively uncommon occurrences in GDM. Possible causes include chronic hypertension and maternal vascular disease (35).

SUMMARY

Normal physiological changes in pregnancy affect nutrient metabolism and insulin resistance. The pathophysiology of GDM is unclear and continues to be an area of research. What is generally known is that maternal hyperglycemia can result from an increase in insulin resistance and/or the inability to increase insulin production to meet the demands of pregnancy. Glucose is the primary nutrient affecting glycemic levels; amino acids and lipids also affect fetal growth and development.

Fetal macrosomia, the most common complication associated with GDM, is associated with maternal hyperglycemia, which in turn possibly causes fetal hyperglycemia and hyperinsulinemia. The goal is to maintain maternal blood glucose levels to within near-normal limits, to decrease the risks associated with GDM.

REFERENCES

1. Deska Pagana K, Pagana TJ. *Mosby's Manual of Diagnostic and Laboratory Tests.* 2nd ed. St. Louis, Mo: Mosby; 2002.

2. Sacher RA, McPherson RA. *Widmann's Clinical Interpretation of Laboratory Tests.* 11th ed. Philadelphia, Pa: FA Davis; 2000.

3. National Cholesterol Education Program. Third Report of the Expert Panel on Detection, Evaluation, and Treatment of High Blood Cholesterol in Adults (Adult Treatment Panel III) Executive Summary. Available at: http://www.nhlbi.nih.gov/guidelines/cholesterol/atp_iii.htm. Accessed December 9, 2004.

4. Moore TR. Diabetes in pregnancy. In: Creasy RK, Resnik R, Iams JD, eds. *Maternal-Fetal Medicine: Principles and Practice.* 5th ed. Philadelphia, Pa: Saunders; 2004:1023–1061.

5. Jansen C, Greenspoon JS, Palmer SM. Diabetes mellitus and pregnancy. In: DeCherney AH, Nathan L, eds. *Current Obstetric and Gynecologic Diagnosis and Treatment.* New York, NY: Lange Medical Books/McGraw-Hill; 2003.

6. Metzger BE, Phelps RL, Dooley SL. The mother in pregnancies complicated by diabetes mellitus. In: Porte JD, Sherwin RS, Baron A, eds. *Ellenberg and Rifkin's Diabetes Mellitus.* 6th ed. New York, NY: McGraw Hill; 2003:619–651.

7. Dickinson JE, Palmer SM. Gestational diabetes: pathophysiology and diagnosis. *Semin Perinatol.* 1990;14:2–11.

8. Buchanan TA, Coustan DR. Diabetes mellitus. In: Burrow GN, Ferris TF, eds. *Medical Complications During Pregnancy.* 4th ed. Philadelphia, Pa: WB Saunders; 1995:29–61.

9. Frienkel N. Banting Lecture 1980: Of pregnancy and progeny. *Diabetes.* 1980;29:1028–1035.

10. Illsley NP. Placental glucose transport in diabetic pregnancy. *Clin Obstet Gynecol.* 2000;43:116–126.

11. Buchanan TA. Effects of maternal diabetes on intrauterine development. In: LeRoith D, Taylor SI, Olefsky JM, eds. *Diabetes Mellitus: A Fundamental and Clinical Text.* 2nd ed. Philadelphia, Pa: Lippincott Williams & Wilkins; 2000:852–862.

12. Landon MB, Catalano PM, Gabbe SG. Diabetes mellitus. In: Gabbe SG, Niebyl JR, Simpson JL, eds. *Obstetrics: Normal and Problem Pregnancies.* Philadelphia, Pa: Churchill Livingstone; 2002:1081–1116.

13. Yamashita H, Jianhua S, Friedman JE. Physiologic and molecular alterations in carbohydrate metabolism during pregnancy and gestational diabetes. *Clin Obstet Gynecol.* 2000;43:87–98.

14. Kuhl C. Etiology and pathogenesis of gestational diabetes. *Diabetes Care.* 1998;21(Suppl 2):B19–B26.

15. Metzger BE, Phelps RL, Dooley SL. The mother in pregnancies complicated by diabetes mellitus. In: Porte D, Sherwin RS, eds. *Ellenberg and Rifkin's Diabetes Mellitus.* 5th ed. Stamford, Conn: Appleton and Lange; 1997:887–955.

16. Sweeney AT, Brown FM. Gestational diabetes mellitus. *Clin Lab Med.* 2001;21:173–192.

17. Kuhl C, Hornnes PJ, Andersen O. Etiology and pathophysiology of gestational diabetes mellitus. *Diabetes.* 1985;34(Suppl 2):S66–S70.

18. Landon MB, Gabbe SG. Diabetes mellitus. In: Barron WM, Lindheimer MD, eds. *Medical Disorders in Pregnancy.* St. Louis, Mo: Mosby; 2000:71–100.

19. Sivan E, Boden G. Free fatty acids, insulin resistance, and pregnancy. *Curr Diab Rep.* 2003;3:319–322.

20. Knopp RH, Bergelin RO, Wahl PW, Walden CE. Relationships of infant birth size to maternal lipoproteins, apoproteins, fuels, hormones, clinical chemistries, and body weight at 36 weeks' gestation. *Diabetes.* 1985;34(Suppl 2):S71–S77.

21. Elster N. Less is more: the risks of multiple births. *Fertil Steril.* 2000;74:617–623.

22. Corrado F, Caputo F, Facciola G, Mancuso A. Gestational glucose intolerance in multiple pregnancy. *Diabetes Care.* 2003;26:1646.

23. Pinborg A, Loft A, Schmidt L, Langhoff-Roos J, Andersen AN. Maternal risks and perinatal outcome in a Danish national cohort of 1005 twin pregnancies: the role of in vitro fertilization. *Acta Obstet Gynecol Scand.* 2004;83:75–84.

24. Fitzsimmons BP, Bebbington MW, Fluker MR. Perinatal and neonatal outcomes in multiple gestations: assisted reproduction versus spontaneous conception. *Am J Obstet Gynecol.* 1998; 179:1162–1167.

25. Buhling KJ, Henrich W, Starr E, Lubke M, Bertran S, Siebert G, Dudenhausen JW. Risk for gestational diabetes and hypertension for women with twin pregnancy compared to singleton pregnancy. *Arch Gynecol Obstet.* 2003;269:33–36.

26. Wein P, Warwick MM, Beischer NA. Gestational diabetes in twin pregnancy: prevalence and long-term implications. *Aust N Z J Obstet Gynaecol.* 1992;32:325–327.

27. Henderson CE, Scarpelli S, LaRosa D, Divon MY. Assessing the risk of gestational diabetes in twin gestation. *J Nat Med Assoc.* 1995;87:757–758.

28. Moses RG, Webb AJ, Lucas EM, Davis WS. Twin pregnancy outcomes for women with gestational diabetes mellitus compared with glucose tolerant women. *Aust N Z J Obstet Gynaecol.* 2003;43:38–40.

29. Dwyer PL, Oats JN, Walstab JE, Beischer NA. Glucose tolerance in twin pregnancy. *Aust N Z J Obstet Gynaecol.* 1982;22:131–134.

30. Roach VJ, Lau TK, Wilson D, Rogers MS. The incidence of gestational diabetes in multiple pregnancy. *Aust N Z J Obstet Gynaecol.* 1998;38:56–57.

31. Mestman JH. Interaction between pregnancy, gestational diabetes, and long-term maternal outcome. In: Reece EA, Coustan DR, Gabbe SG, eds. *Diabetes in Women: Adolescence, Pregnancy and Menopause.* Philadelphia, Pa: Lippincott, Williams & Wilkins; 2004:233–242.

32. Kalkoff RK. Impact of maternal fuels and nutritional state on fetal growth. *Diabetes.* 1991; 40(Suppl 2):S61-S65.

33. Health and Administration Development Group. *Diabetes Management: Clinical Pathways, Guidelines and Patient Education.* Gaithersburg, Md: Aspen Publications; 1999.

34. Pedersen J. *The Pregnant Diabetic and Her Newborn.* 2nd ed. Baltimore, Md: Williams & Wilkins; 1977.

35. Galan HL, Battaglia FC. The biology of normal and abnormal fetal growth and development. In: Reece EA, Coustan DR, Gabbe SG, eds. *Diabetes in Women: Adolescence, Pregnancy and Menopause.* Philadelphia, Pa: Lippincott, Williams & Wilkins; 2004:159–168.

Classification, Screening, and Diagnosis

Alyce M. Thomas, RD

OBJECTIVES   After completing this chapter, you will be able to do the following:

1. Summarize the various classifications of diabetes during pregnancy.
2. Outline the risk factors associated with gestational diabetes mellitus (GDM).
3. Describe the differences between the glucose challenge test (GCT) and the oral glucose tolerance test (OGTT).
4. Compare the threshold glucose values of the American Diabetes Association and the World Health Organization (WHO) in the diagnosis of GDM.
5. Evaluate the results of the blood glucose level using the current recommended criteria for screening and diagnosing GDM.

CLASSIFICATION OF DIABETES IN PREGNANCY

Several systems have been developed to identify the various types of diabetes during pregnancy. One of the earliest classification systems was developed by White, from the Joslin Diabetes Center, in 1949 (1). White's system was based on the following criteria that affect pregnancy outcome:

- Age at onset of the diabetes
- Duration of the disease
- Severity of vascular complications

The White classification was modified through the years to include GDM (2). For a description of each classification, see Table 3.1 (2).

TABLE 3.1 Modified White Classification of Diabetes in Pregnancy

Class	Description
A_1	Glucose tolerance test abnormal. No symptoms. Blood glucose levels are maintained by medical nutrition therapy only.
A_2	Glucose tolerance test abnormal and insulin is required to maintain normal levels.
B	Onset ≥20 years of age and relatively short duration (<10 y).
C	Relatively young onset (age 10–19 y) or relatively long duration (10–19 y).
D	Very young onset (<10 y of age) or very long duration (≥20 y) or evidence of minimal vascular disease (benign retinopathy).
F	Renal disease (nephropathy).
R	Proliferative retinopathy.
H	Arteriosclerotic heart disease.
T	Pregnancy after renal transplantation.

Source: Data are from reference 2.

TABLE 3.2 Hollingsworth Classification of Glucose Intolerance in Pregnancy

Type	Clinical Features
Type 1	Ketosis-prone, insulin-dependent due to islet cell loss, diagnosed before pregnancy
Type 2	Ketosis-resistant, non-insulin-dependent, insulin-resistant, obesity, family history, and age are common factors
Type 3 or gestational diabetes	Occurs only in pregnancy
Type 4 or secondary diabetes	Associated with endocrine disorders

Source: Data are from reference 4.

In 1979, the National Diabetes Data Group devised a simple classification of diabetes, which distinguished type 1 from type 2 (3). Hollingsworth adapted this classification for use during pregnancy; Hollingsworth's classification can be found in Table 3.2 (4).

In 1995, Buchanan and Coustan (5) classified diabetes affecting pregnant women into two large groups: pregestational and gestational diabetes. Their classification was based on when the diabetes developed during the pregnancy, metabolic control and timing, and the presence of maternal vascular and medical complications. There are, however, physicians who continue to use the White classification because it specifies the risk of the severity of maternal and fetal complications during pregnancy. The major drawbacks to the White classification are that it does not address glycemic control and it does not differentiate between type 1 and type 2 diabetes in women before they conceive (6).

SCREENING

Risk Factors

The position of the American Diabetes Association is to assess every pregnant woman for risk of GDM at her first prenatal visit (7,8). This is also the recommendation of ACOG (9). The risk factors are divided into three categories (10): low risk, high risk, and average risk.

Low Risk

Women classified as low risk if they meet all of the following criteria (8):

- Younger than 25 years of age
- No personal history of glucose intolerance or diabetes
- Normal prepregnancy body mass index (BMI) (<25.0)
- No family history of diabetes in a first-degree relative
- No history of poor obstetrical outcome
- Not a member of an ethnic group with a high prevalence of gestational diabetes

According to American Diabetes Association criteria (8), low-risk women do not require glucose testing.

High Risk

A woman is considered high risk if she meets one or more of the following criteria (8):

- History of GDM
- Obesity (BMI > 30.0)
- Glycosuria
- Strong family history of diabetes
- Prior poor obstetrical outcome (ie, stillbirth, birth defects)
- Member of a high-risk ethnic group (Hispanic, African, Native American, South or East Asian, or Pacific Islands ancestry)

Women identified at high risk for developing GDM must undergo glucose testing at their initial prenatal visit. If the test results are negative, they are retested at 24 to 28 weeks of pregnancy (8).

Average Risk

Women who do not fit the first two categories are considered at average risk. These women are tested at 24 to 28 weeks of gestation (8).

Socioeconomic Factors

Social and economic factors also play a role in the risk of diabetes. Women with GDM are more likely to have lower income and educational levels, to be uninsured, and to lack access to health care (11). A lower socioeconomic status is associated with a higher incidence of morbidity and mortality (11).

Criteria and Approaches

Currently, there is no agreement within the international community on the glucose levels used to screen for and diagnose GDM. The American Diabetes Association and WHO use different criteria to diagnose gestational diabetes. WHO defines GDM as the joint category of diabetes (fasting glucose $\geq$ 7.0 mmol/L [126 mg/dL] or 2-hour glucose $\geq$ 11.1 mmol/L [200 mg/dL]) and impaired glucose tolerance (IGT) (2-hour glucose > 7.8 mmol/L [140 mg/dL]) and not diabetes (12).

The American Diabetes Association recommends either a one- or two-step approach to screening and diagnosis (7,8). In the one-step approach, the woman is given a 75-g OGTT without a prior plasma glucose screen. This approach is considered cost effective and is recommended for use in a high-risk population (7,8). The two-step approach uses the GCT and the OGTT (8). In the GCT, the woman is given a 50-g oral glucose load as a screen, and the plasma or serum glucose levels are measured in 1 hour. The test is given regardless to the time of day or if food was consumed before the test was administered. Fasting before this test may result in a false-negative result (13). The woman is instructed not to smoke, eat, or participate in any physical activity during the testing time (8). If the results of the test exceed the threshold of 140 mg/dL (7.8 mmol/L), the 3-hour OGTT with 100 g is performed. Approximately 80% of women with GDM will be identified if 140 mg/dL (7.8 mmol/L) is used as the cutoff value. If 130 mg/dL (7.2 mmol/L) is used as the threshold, then 90% of women with GDM will be identified (8). For a screening and diagnosis flowchart using 140 mg/dL (7.8 mmol/L) as the cutoff value, see Figure 3.1 (14).

The specificity of the GCT is 100% and 90%, for thresholds of 130 mg/dL (7.2 mmol/L) and 140 mg/dL (7.8 mmol/L), respectively. The sensitivity of this test is 78% at 140 mg/dL (7.8 mmol/L) and 87% at 130 mg/dL (7.2 mmol/L) (7,15). A screening threshold of 130 mg/dL (7.2 mmol/L) or 140 mg/dL (7.8 mmol/L) is deemed accept-

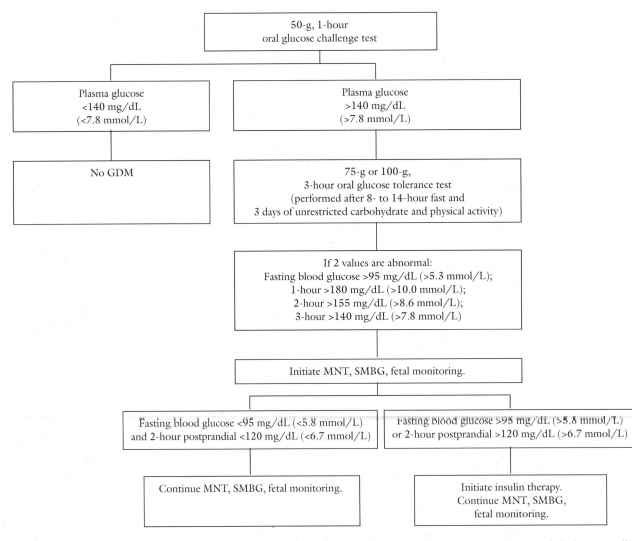

FIGURE 3.1. Screening and diagnosis of gestational diabetes. Abbreviations: GDM, gestational diabetes mellitus; MNT, medical nutrition therapy; SMBG, self-monitoring of blood glucose. Adapted from: Jovanovic L, ed. *Medical Management of Pregnancy Complicated by Diabetes.* 3rd ed. Alexandria, Va. American Diabetes Association; 2000. Used with permission.

able by ACOG (9). A random blood glucose level of ≥200 mg/dL (11.1 mmol/L) is considered a diagnosis of GDM, if confirmed on a subsequent day (8). Glucose meters are not used in screening for GDM, although Buhling et al found the accuracy of certain meters within the range of laboratory results (16). Others have suggested using the fasting plasma glucose as a cost-effective method for screening for GDM (17–20).

WHO uses the 75 g, 2 hour OGTT as a diagnostic test in women considered at high risk for GDM. The high-risk group includes older women, those with a previous history of glucose intolerance, women with a history of large-for-gestational-age babies, women from high-risk ethnic groups, and all pregnant women with elevated fasting or casual blood glucose levels (12).

The Debate Over Universal Screening

The utility of universal screening for diabetes in pregnancy is a controversial subject (21,22). Before the Fourth International Workshop-Conference on Gestational Diabetes made its recommendations, all pregnant women in the United States were screened for GDM (23). ACOG previously recommended screening all women older than 30 years; younger women would be screened if one or more risk factors was present (24). Most of the controversy stems from the lack of data from well-controlled studies to determine the ideal screening criteria. Without clear evidence of its benefits, universal screening is considered by some to be an unnecessary expense (21,25,26).

In 2003, the consensus of the United States Preventive Services Task Force (USPSTF) was that "The evidence is insufficient to recommend for or against routine screening for gestational diabetes and has placed this in the USPSTF Recommendations and Ratings as I" (27). A rating of I finds the service to be lacking, of poor quality, or conflicting, and the balance of benefits and harms cannot be determined. However, the USPSTF found fair to good evidence that screening combined with diet and insulin therapy can reduce the rate of fetal macrosomia in women with GDM. Other outcomes, such as cesarean delivery, birth injury, and neonatal morbidity or mortality, were not found to be substantially reduced. According to the USPSTF, most studies were too small to detect any appreciable changes in outcome. With no evidence-based guidelines for health care providers to follow, the question regarding screening in pregnancy remains unanswered.

For health care providers who support universal screening, the identification of women at risk for future type 2 diabetes is a major reason for testing during pregnancy. Earlier detection may prevent the complications associated with uncontrolled diabetes (28).

The potential adverse effects of maternal diabetes on the offspring of women with GDM must also be considered (29). In a study that compared rates of infant mortality and morbidity with maternal glucose concentration in the third trimester, Pettitt et al found an increase in the incidence of perinatal mortality, macrosomia, preeclampsia, and cesarean sections with an increase in plasma glucose (30). The prevention of macrosomia and the possible risk of shoulder dystocia or other birth injury supports the case for screening all pregnant women for GDM. Selective screening may miss some women with GDM (31,32). A cohort study found that 4% of women diagnosed with GDM would have been missed using the American Diabetes Association's screening criteria (33).

In a Danish study (34) that examined the complications associated with GDM, women with GDM had a higher incidence of lower gestational age at delivery than women without GDM. A study of approximately 9,500 pregnant women in China came to similar conclusions (35). Using the screening criteria of the American Diabetes Association and WHO, 24% and 12%, respectively, of the women confirmed as having GDM in that study would not have been diagnosed (35). An Australian study found no difference in the prevalence of

GDM in women classified as low risk using the WHO criteria for developing GDM from other women with GDM (36). Wong and Tan concluded that the GCT was a useful tool in screening women with no apparent risk factors for GDM (37).

DIAGNOSIS

The OGTT is a diagnostic test in which the woman is given a 100-g glucose load after an overnight fast of 8 to 14 hours, 3 previous days of unrestricted diet of ≥150 g of carbohydrate, and unlimited physical activity. Blood is drawn at fasting, and 1, 2, and 3 hours after ingesting the glucose solution. The woman is instructed not to smoke and to sit for the duration of the test (8). Gestational diabetes is confirmed when two or more values exceed the values described in Table 3.3 (8). The diagnostic criteria are those recommended by the Fourth International Workshop-Conference on Gestational Diabetes Mellitus (38). These values are based on the Carpenter and Coustan (39) modification from the 1979 National Diabetes Data Group (NDDG) (3).

In the 75-g glucose test used by WHO (12), fasting, 1-hour, and 2-hour tests are used to diagnose GDM (see Table 3.4) (8). The diagnosis is made when the fasting glucose is greater than 126 mg/dL (7.0 mmol/L) and the 2-hour glucose is greater than 200 mg/dL (11.1mmol/L) (40). Australia, New Zealand, and most European countries use the WHO criteria.

Abnormal OGTT Values

For women with one abnormal OGTT value, researchers have proposed several different courses of treatment. In a 1989 study by Langer et al (41), women with one abnormal OGTT level were randomized into two groups: treated and untreated. The treated group followed a strict diabetes protocol of diet and insulin, if necessary. The untreated group received no medical nutrition therapy or insulin intervention, and both groups self-monitored their blood glucose levels. A higher incidence of macrosomia and other neonatal complications was found in the untreated group. The authors concluded that women with one abnormal OGTT value should be managed as though they had GDM (41). Other investigators have found higher rates of preterm birth, premature rupture of membranes, or breech presentation in women with impaired glucose tolerance (42–44). The USPSTF recommends retesting the blood glucose at 32 weeks if the GCT is abnormal and the OGTT results are normal (27).

TABLE 3.3 Diagnosis of Gestational Diabetes Mellitus Using 100-g Load

Time	mg/dL	mmol/L
Fasting	95	5.3
1 hour	180	10.0
2 hour	155	8.6
3 hour	140	7.8

Source: Reprinted with permission from American Diabetes Association. Gestational diabetes mellitus. *Diabetes Care*. 2004;27(Suppl 1):S88-S90.

TABLE 3.4 Diagnosis of Gestational Diabetes Mellitus Using 75-g Load

Time	mg/dL	mmol/L
Fasting	95	5.3
1 hour	180	10.0
2 hour	155	8.6

Source: Reprinted with permission from American Diabetes Association. Gestational diabetes mellitus. *Diabetes Care*. 2004;27(Suppl 1):S88-S90.

Criticisms of Oral Glucose Tolerance Tests

Although widely used as the most definitive test in diagnosing gestational diabetes, the OGTT is not without its shortcomings. In a review article, Hanna and Peters list several limitations of the OGTT, including the expense, the time involved, the unpleasant taste, and that it is unrelated to body weight (26).

There is also disagreement with the diagnostic criteria used for gestational diabetes. An Australian study (45) to determine a reference range for women at low risk for gestational diabetes disagreed with the current diagnostic criteria. It recommended that the levels of the OGTT be further decreased to 90 mg/dL (5.0 mmol/L) and 140 mg/dL (7.8 mmol/L) for the fasting glucose and 2-hour levels, respectively (45). Conversely, Rajab and Mehdi (46) have suggested increasing the threshold level from 140 mg/dL (7.8 mmol/L) to 150 mg/dL (8.4 mmol/L), thereby reducing the number of OGTTs performed.

Until large-scale studies are conducted, arguments on the current practice of screening and diagnosing of gestational diabetes will continue. In the meantime, the recommendations of the ACOG (9), which follow the Carpenter-Coustan (39) criteria for the diagnosis of GDM, can be used:

- A screening test consisting of a 50-g, 1-hour GCT at 24 to 28 weeks' gestation.
- The screening test should be performed in a laboratory using plasma glucose.
- Universal screening using the GCT is the most sensitive approach; however, women classified as low risk may not benefit from testing. It is left to the individual clinician to determine the feasibility of testing each pregnant woman.

SUMMARY

In pregnancy, diabetes is classified using the American Diabetes Association criteria, although some health care providers continue to use the White system of classification. The requirement for diabetes screening in pregnancy remains controversial. ACOG recommends screening all pregnant women for gestational diabetes (9). The screening could be the patient's history, clinical risk factors, or a laboratory test. In the past, it was customary to screen for diabetes in pregnancy using the 50-g GCT; currently, this test is not universally performed.

There are also questions about the use of the 75-g or 100-g OGTT for diagnosing GDM. Although most countries use the one-step, 75-g OGTT, the two-step approach (GCT and 100-g OGTT) is most commonly used in the United States to diagnose GDM. Clearly, evidence-based research is needed for more definitive practice guidelines.

REFERENCES

1. White P. Pregnancy complicating diabetes. *Am J Med*. 1949;7:609–616.
2. White P. Classification of obstetric diabetes. *Am J Obstet Gynecol*. 1978;130:228–230.
3. National Diabetes Data Group. Classification and diagnosis of diabetes mellitus and other categories of glucose intolerance. *Diabetes*. 1979;28:1039–1057.
4. Hollingsworth DR. *Pregnancy, Diabetes and Birth: A Management Guide*. 2nd ed. Baltimore, Md: Williams & Wilkins; 1992.
5. Buchanan TA, Coustan DR. Diabetes mellitus. In: Burrow GN, Ferris TF, eds. *Medical Complications in Pregnancy*. 4th ed. Philadelphia, Pa: WB Saunders; 1995:29–61.
6. Franz MJ, ed. *Diabetes in the Life Cycle and Research: A Core Curriculum for Diabetes Education*. 5th ed. Chicago, Ill: American Association of Diabetes Educators; 2003.

7. American Diabetes Association. Diagnosis and classification of diabetes mellitus. *Diabetes Care.* 2004;27(Suppl 1):S5–S10.

8. American Diabetes Association. Gestational diabetes mellitus. *Diabetes Care.* 2004;27(Suppl 1):S88–S90.

9. American College of Obstetricians and Gynecologists Committee on Practice Bulletins—Obstetrics. ACOG Practice Bulletin. Clinical management guidelines for obstetrician-gynecologists. Number 30, September 2001 (replaces Technical Bulletin Number 200, December 1994). Gestational diabetes. *Obstet Gynecol.* 2001;98:525–538.

10. Moore TR. Diabetes in pregnancy. In: Creasy RK, Resnik R. eds. *Maternal-Fetal Medicine: Principles and Practice.* Philadelphia, Pa: Saunders; 2004:1023–1061.

11. Anderson NB, Armstrong CA. Toward understanding the association of socioeconomic status and health: a new challenge for the biophysical approach. *Psychosom Med.* 1995;57:213–225.

12. World Health Organization. *Diabetes Mellitus.* Geneva, Switzerland: World Health Organization, 1985. Tech report series 727.

13. Sermer M, Naylor CD, Gare DJ, Kenshole AB, Ritchie JW, Farine D, Cohen HR, McArthur K, Holzapfel S, Biringer A, Chen E. Impact of increasing carbohydrate intolerance on maternal-fetal outcomes in 3637 women without gestational diabetes: the Toronto Tri-Hospital Gestational Diabetes Project. *Am J Obstet Gynecol.* 1995;173:146–156.

14. Jovanovic L, ed. *Medical Management of Pregnancy Complicated by Diabetes.* 3rd ed. Alexandria, Va. American Diabetes Association; 2000.

15. Rollins G. Updated guidelines outline options for gestational diabetes mellitus. *Rep Med Guidel Outcomes Res.* 2001;12:8–10.

16. Buhling KJ, Henrich W, Kjos SL, Siebert G, Starr E, Dreweck C, Stein U, Dudenhausen JW. Comparison of point-of-care glucose with standard laboratory measurement of the 50g-glucose-challenge test (GCT) during pregnancy. *Clin Biochem.* 2003;36:333–337.

17. de Aguiar LG, de Matos HJ, de Brito Gomes M. Could fasting plasma glucose be used for screening high-risk outpatients for gestational diabetes mellitus? *Diabetes Care.* 2001;24:954–955.

18. Perruchini D, Fischer U, Spinas GA, Huch R, Huch A, Lehmann R. Using fasting plasma glucose to screen for gestational diabetes mellitus: prospective population based study. *BMJ.* 1999;319:812–815.

19. Reichelt AJ, Spichler ER, Branchtein L, Nucci LB, Franco LJ, Schmidt MI. Fasting plasma glucose is a useful test for the detection of gestational diabetes. Brazilian Study of Gestational Diabetes (EBDG) Working Group. *Diabetes Care.* 1998;21:1246–1249.

20. Tam WH, Rogers MS, Yip SK, Lau TK, Leung TY. Which screening test is the best for gestational impaired glucose tolerance and gestational diabetes mellitus? *Diabetes Care.* 2000;23:1432.

21. Jarrett RJ, Castro-Soares J, Dornhorst A, Beard RW, Castro-Soares J. Should we screen for gestational diabetes? *BMJ.* 1997;315:736–739.

22. Agarwal MM, Punnose J. Gestational diabetes: implications of variation in diagnostic criteria. *Int J Gynaecol Obstet.* 2002;78:45–46.

23. Lehmann J. Screening, diagnosis and education of women with gestational diabetes. *Aust J Adv Nurs.* 1992;10:14–20.

24. Coustan DR. Making the diagnosis of gestational diabetes mellitus. *Clin Obstet Gynecol.* 2000;43:99–105.

25. Wen SW, Liu S, Kramer MS, Joseph KS, Levitt C, Marcoux S, Liston RM. Impact of prenatal glucose screening on the diagnosis of gestational diabetes and on pregnancy outcomes. *Am J Epidemiol.* 2000;152:1009–1014.

26. Hanna FW, Peters JR. Screening for gestational diabetes; past, present and future. *Diabet Med.* 2002;19:351–358.

27. US Preventive Services Task Force (USPTF). Screening for gestational diabetes mellitus: recommendation and rationale. *Am Fam Physician.* 2003;68:331–335.

28. Bartha JL, Martinez-Del-Fresno P, Comino-Delgado R. Gestational diabetes mellitus diagnosed during early pregnancy. *Am J Obstet Gynecol.* 2000;182:346–350.

29. Ardawi MS, Nasrat HA, Jamal HS, Al-Sagaaf HM, Mustafa BE. Screening for gestational diabetes mellitus in pregnant females. *Saudi Med J.* 2000;21:155–160.

30. Pettitt DJ, Knowler WC, Baird HR, Bennett PH. Gestational diabetes: infant and maternal complications of pregnancy in relation to third-trimester glucose tolerance in the Pima Indians. *Diabetes Care.* 1980;3:458–464.

31. Jovanovic L. Controversies in the diagnosis and treatment of gestational diabetes. *Cleve Clin J Med.* 2000;67:481–482, 485–486, 488.

32. Pettitt DJ. Gestational diabetes mellitus: who to test. How to test. *Diabetes Care.* 1998;21:1789.

33. Ricart W, Bach C, Fernandez-Real JM, Biarnes J, Sabria J. Impact of selective screening for gestational diabetes in a Spanish population. *Medical Clinics (Barc).* 1999;113:331–333.

34. Svare JA, Hansen BB, Molsted-Pedersen L. Perinatal complications in women with gestational diabetes mellitus. *Acta Obstet Gynecol Scand.* 2001;80:899–904.

35. Yang X, Hsu-Hage B, Yu L, Simmons D. Selective screening for gestational diabetes in Chinese women. *Diabetes Care.* 2002;25:796.

36. Moses RG, Moses J, Davis WS. Gestational diabetes: do lean young Caucasian women need to be tested? *Diabetes Care.* 1998;21:1803–1806.

37. Wong L, Tan AS. The glucose challenge test for screening gestational diabetes in pregnant women with no risk factors. *Singapore Med J.* 2001;42:517–521.

38. Metzer BE, Coustan DR. Summary and recommendations of the Fourth International Workshop-Conference on Gestational Diabetes Mellitus. *Diabetes Care.* 1998;21(Suppl 2):B161–167.

39. Carpenter MW, Coustan DR. Criteria screening tests for gestational diabetes. *Am J Obstet Gynecol.* 1982;144:768–773.

40. Schmidt MI, Matos MC, Reichelt AJ, Forti AC, de Lima L, Duncan BB. Prevalence of gestational diabetes mellitus-do the new WHO criteria make a difference? Brazilian Gestational Diabetes Study Group. *Diabet Med.* 2000;17:376–380.

41. Langer O, Anyaegbunam A, Brustman L, Divon M. Management of women with one abnormal oral glucose tolerance test value reduces adverse outcome in pregnancy. *Am J Obstet Gynecol.* 1989;161:593–599.

42. Yang X, Hsu-Hage B, Zhang H, Zhang C, Zhang Y, Zhang C. Women with impaired glucose tolerance during pregnancy have significantly poor pregnancy outcomes. *Diabetes Care.* 2002;25:1619–1624.

43. Ostlund I, Hanson U, Bjorklund A, Hjertberg R, Eva N, Nordlander E, Swahn ML, Wager J. Maternal and fetal outcomes if gestational impaired glucose tolerance is not treated. *Diabetes Care.* 2003;26:2107–2111.

44. Yang X, Hsu-Hage B, Dong L, Shao P, Wang H, Tian H, Chen Y, Zhang H. Intensive diabetes management may improve pregnancy; outcomes in Chinese gravidas with impaired glucose tolerance. *Diabetes Care.* 2003;26:254–255.

45. Moses RG, Moses M, Russell KG, Schier GM. The 75-g glucose tolerance test in pregnancy: a reference range determined on a low-risk population and related to selected pregnancy outcomes. *Diabetes Care.* 1998;21:1807–1811.

46. Rajab KE, Mehdi S. Pregnancy outcome among gestational diabetics with blood glucose levels between 7.7 and 8.3 mmol/L. *Int J Gynaecol Obstet.* 1998;63:59–61.

4

Maternal and Fetal Complications Associated with Gestational Diabetes Mellitus

Alyce M. Thomas, RD, and Yolanda M. Gutierrez, MS, PhD, RD

OBJECTIVES

After completing this chapter, you will be able to do the following:

1. Describe four maternal complications that may complicate gestational diabetes mellitus (GDM).
2. Discuss the fetal complications associated with GDM.

OVERVIEW

GDM is associated with a higher incidence of maternal and fetal complications. The maternal complications include hypertensive disorders of pregnancy, polyhydramnios, and higher rates of preterm deliveries and cesarean sections (1–3). Fetal complications include macrosomia, preterm birth, neonatal hypoglycemia, hypocalcemia, hyperbilirubinemia, hypomagnesemia, polycythemia, respiratory distress syndrome, and increased rate of stillbirth (4). Although rarely seen in GDM, congenital anomalies may occur if GDM is diagnosed in the early first trimester (4).

MATERNAL COMPLICATIONS

Hypertension

Classification

Hypertension is a complication that could antedate or develop during pregnancy. The classification created by the Working Group of the National High Blood Pressure Education Program (5) identifies the following types of hypertension in pregnancy:

1. *Preeclampsia.* A pregnancy-specific syndrome that is usually observed after the 20th week of pregnancy, preeclampsia is defined by (*a*) a systolic blood pressure >140 mm Hg or a diastolic blood pressure ≥90 mm Hg in a woman who was normotensive before pregnancy, and (*b*) proteinuria. In the absence of proteinuria, preeclampsia may be suspected if the elevated blood pressure is accompanied by headache, blurred vision, and abdominal pain, or by abnormal liver enzymes and low platelet counts. The blood pressure usually returns to baseline within days to weeks after delivery (5).

2. *Eclampsia.* Eclampsia is the occurrence in a woman with preeclampsia of seizures that cannot be attributed to other causes (5,6).

3. *Chronic hypertension.* This is defined as hypertension (systolic ≥140 mm Hg or diastolic ≥90 mm Hg) diagnosed before the 20th week of pregnancy. This category also includes hypertension that is diagnosed for the first time during pregnancy and that does not resolve postpartum.

4. *Preeclampsia superimposed on chronic hypertension.* This is preeclampsia that occurs in women with hypertension. Superimposed preeclampsia may be suspected from the following (5,6):
   - Hypertension and proteinuria before 20 weeks' gestation
   - A sudden increase in proteinuria
   - A sudden increase in blood pressure in a woman whose hypertension was previously well controlled
   - Thrombocytopenia (platelet count < 100,000 cells/mm^3)

5. *Gestational hypertension.* Defined as a blood pressure elevation detected for the first time after midpregnancy, gestational hypertension is distinguished from preeclampsia by the absence of proteinuria. If proteinuria develops and hypertension returns to normal by the 12th week postpartum, the diagnosis is changed to preeclampsia. If the blood pressure remains elevated following delivery, then the woman is diagnosed as having chronic hypertension (5).

Outcomes

Hypertension in pregnancy is associated with outcomes that range from favorable to poor, depending on the classification. Women with mild to moderate chronic hypertension usually have good outcomes (5–7). If chronic hypertension is superimposed with preeclampsia or if eclampsia develops, the risk of an unfavorable outcome increases (5–7). Preeclampsia is a major cause of maternal and/or fetal morbidity and mortality. The complications associated with preeclampsia include placental abruption, cerebral hemorrhage, pulmonary edema, acute renal failure, and liver infarction (6,7). A potentially fatal form of preeclampsia, the HELLP Syndrome (*h*emolytic anemia, *e*levated *l*iver enzymes, and *l*ow *p*latelets), is characterized by liver dysfunction and coagulation abnormalities (6).

Treatment

The treatment for hypertension in GDM is the same as the treatment for hypertension in pregnancy without GDM. It may include medication, medical nutrition therapy, and, in certain cases, hospitalization (6–8). Although sodium is not routinely restricted in pregnancy, a low-sodium diet may be indicated if the woman with chronic hypertension followed this regimen before conception (6–8). The use of dietary calcium, magnesium, and zinc in the management of hypertensive disorders in pregnancy has yielded conflicting results (6–12).

Incidence

Although it has been suggested that the incidence of chronic hypertension is increased in GDM, there are no studies that show a direct correlation. Some researchers found a higher incidence of hypertension in women with GDM compared with women with normal glucose tolerance (13–15). The severity of the maternal glycemic level is a possible predictive factor of hypertension in pregnancy (16,17). Other researchers found no difference in the incidence of hypertension in women with GDM when compared with women with normal pregnancies (18,19).

Polyhydramnios

The amniotic fluid index is the sum of the measurements of the vertical depth of amniotic fluid in each of the four quadrants of the amniotic cavity and depends on the week of gestation (20). Polyhydramnios is more often seen in pregnancies with fetal complications, such as congenital anomalies, than in normal pregnancies. If the amniotic fluid index in polyhydramnios exceeds 200 mm, this could be a result of poor maternal glycemic control, leading to an increase in fetal urination and amniotic fluid (21). Polyhydramnios is often associated with congenital anomalies of the central nervous system or gastrointestinal tract.

Preterm Delivery and Cesarean Sections

A delivery that occurs before 38 weeks' gestation is considered preterm (22). Maternal complications associated with preterm delivery include preeclampsia, a decrease in maternal renal function, and maternal hyperglycemia (22,23). Early delivery is not indicated in GDM if there are no complications during the pregnancy. It may be necessary to induce labor if the fetal weight is estimated to be large for gestational age or to reduce the risk of birth trauma. An amniocentesis will confirm fetal lung maturity if the gestational age is less than 38 weeks (22,24).

Women with GDM are at increased risk for cesarean sections caused by a higher incidence of maternal complications, such as macrosomia, fetal distress, or failed induction (1,25–27). The health care provider may recommend a cesarean delivery, to decrease the risk of maternal mortality and morbidity (21).

Other Maternal Complications

Certain conditions, such as nephropathy, retinopathy, and coronary artery disease, are more commonly associated with preexisting diabetes mellitus than with GDM. A woman diagnosed with GDM in the early first trimester could have unrecognized type 1 or type 2 diabetes and could present with these complications (24,25).

FETAL COMPLICATIONS

The incidence of fetal complications in women with GDM is lower than in women with preexisting diabetes but higher than in women with normal pregnancies (26,27). Although GDM is defined as diabetes first recognized in the current pregnancy, it may be reasonable to assume that the woman diagnosed with diabetes in the first or early second trimester may have developed this condition before pregnancy. If so, the fetus is at risk for developing congenital anomalies. The fetal outcome may be immediate (eg, macrosomia, hypoglycemia, hypocalcemia, respiratory distress syndrome) or long term (obesity and type 2 diabetes later in life or poor neurologic development) (28–33).

Macrosomia

The incidence of macrosomia has increased in the United States and other developed countries (34,35). It is the most common fetal complication associated with GDM, with a prevalence rate of 15% to 45% (1,26).

There is considerable variation in the literature regarding the minimum weight (eg, 4,000 g, 4,100 g, 4,500 g, or 4,586 g) used to define macrosomia. The American College of Obstetricians and Gynecologists (ACOG) defines fetal macrosomia as a birth weight of more than 4,500 g, irrespective of gestational age or other demographic variables (36). Some researchers use different cutoffs for patients with or without diabetes (37).

A three-step definition for macrosomia proposed by Boulet et al incorporates easily remembered birth-weight cutoff values, which may facilitate assessing risk and predicting outcome (38):

1. Grade 1 macrosomia is defined as a birth weight between 4,000 and 4,499 g. This definition may be useful in the identification of increased risks of labor and newborn complications.
2. Grade 2 macrosomia indicates a birth weight between 4,500 and 4,999 g. This grade may be predictive of neonatal morbidity.
3. Grade 3 macrosomia indicates a birth weight greater than 5,000 g. This may be a stronger indicator of infant morbidity or mortality risk than grade 2.

Boulet et al also demonstrated that mothers of the macrosomic infants were more likely to have maternal complications, including diabetes and hypertension, than women of normosomic infants (38). Macrosomic infants were at a greater risk of being delivered by cesarean section and of birth injury than were nonmacrosomic infants.

Fetal exposure to high maternal plasma concentrations of glucose is the underlying cause of macrosomia. In a study by Jimenez-Moleon et al, GDM was associated with a greater incidence of fetal macrosomia (39). In response to this excessive transport of glucose across the placenta barrier, large amounts of insulin are produced by the fetal pancreas. Insulin is a growth hormone, and an increased secretion will result in excessive adipose tissue deposits in the fetus, primarily in the organs, chest, and abdominal area (40). The fetal head becomes large with this change in body composition, and a corresponding increase in the shoulder and abdominal areas causes birth to be more difficult. There is an increased incidence of shoulder dystocia in babies whose mothers have GDM. Shoulder dystocia increases the risk of injury to the fetal head and neck, including brachial plexus injury, Erb-Duchenne paralysis, and asphyxia (41). Other factors affecting fetal weight include the concentration of maternal plasma amino acids and free fatty acids (42–44).

Additional investigation of the relationship between the prevalence of documented risk factors (such as maternal obesity and diabetes mellitus) and changes in the incidence of macrosomia is warranted. It must also be determined whether clinical interventions to treat women with specific risk factors are effective in preventing macrosomia.

Neonatal Hypoglycemia

Neonatal hypoglycemia occurs shortly after birth when the infant is no longer receiving a continuous supply of maternal glucose (45). High levels of insulin will continue to be produced by the infant when the umbilical cord is clamped. The normal glucose level of the neonate is 40 to 120 mg/dL (46). Without the supply of glucose from its mother, the glycemic levels of the infant will drop rapidly. The neonate's glucose level may drop to 40 mg/dL or below in the first 12 hours of life. To avoid hypoglycemia, early initiation of oral feedings with breastmilk and frequent blood glucose monitoring are recommended. If the neonate's glycemic levels remain below normal, then intravenous glucose will be necessary. The risks associated with neonatal hypoglycemia are seizures, cerebral damage, and death (46,47).

Respiratory Distress Syndrome

The risk of respiratory distress syndrome in the infant whose mother has GDM is higher than it is in the infant whose mother has a normal pregnancy (21). The respiratory system is the last organ to mature in the fetus (48). Fetal lung maturity may be delayed when women have pregnancies with poor glycemic control (49). Fetal hyperinsulinemia may interfere with phosphatidyl glycerol (PG) by decreasing the amount necessary for the production of surfactant. Measuring the PG level is the most sensitive indicator of lung maturation and adequate surfactant. This test is usually not performed if there are no complications and the diabetes is well controlled during the pregnancy (50).

Neonatal Hypocalcemia

Neonatal hypocalcemia occurs when the infant's serum calcium level is less than 7 mg/dL (51). During pregnancy, calcium, magnesium, and other minerals are transported from the mother to the fetus. In the normal neonate, the parathyroid hormone and vitamin D are stimulated into action when the serum calcium decreases. However, in GDM, there is a reduction in the levels of magnesium and parathyroid hormone (52). This in turn may cause fetal hypomagnesemia and may lead to lower levels of fetal parathyroid hormone and eventually to neonatal hypocalcemia (21,32,52). Infants born with hypocalcemia may be jittery or cyanotic, have feeding problems, or develop seizures. The treatment for hypocalcemia is an infusion of 10% calcium gluconate. If hypomagnesemia is present, the treatment will consist of correcting the magnesium levels before the calcium (47,52).

Neonatal Hyperbilirubinemia

Hyperbilirubinemia in a neonate is defined as a serum bilirubin greater than 13 mg/dL (53). The risk of neonatal jaundice in pregnancies complicated by GDM is 20%, vs 10% in normal pregnancies (21). The pathogenesis of hyperbilirubinemia is not well understood, although what is known that it is associated with an increase in red blood cell production or newborn hemoglobin catabolism. The treatment for hyperbilirubinemia is phototherapy or exchange transfusion (21,47).

Polycythemia

Polycythemia is an abnormal hematocrit of greater than 65% (47,54). The exact mechanism is unknown, but polycythemia may result from an increase in the red cell production in response to a decrease in available oxygen to the fetus (21). Fetal hypoxia occurring in the presence of fetal hyperinsulinemia can increase oxygen consumption and cardiac load as a result of poor maternal glycemic control (20,54). A higher incidence of polycythemia is found in the infants of women with GDM. The therapy for polycythemia is a partial exchange transfusion, to decrease the red blood cell mass (47,54).

Congenital Anomalies

Congenital anomalies are more common in infants whose mothers have preexisting diabetes than in those whose mothers have GDM (45,54). Poor glycemic control during the critical period of organogenesis could attribute to the higher rate of malformations. While the incidence of congenital anomalies in infants of women with GDM is the same as for infants of pregnant women without GDM, the rate of congenital malformations could increase if GDM were diagnosed in the early first trimester (47). The anomalies may affect the cardiovascular, central nervous, skeletal, genitourinary, and gastrointestinal systems of the fetus.

SUMMARY

Maternal complications associated with GDM include hypertensive disorders, polyhydramnios, difficult birth, preterm delivery, and a higher rate of cesarean sections. Fetal and neonatal complications include macrosomia, hypoglycemia, respiratory distress syndrome, hypocalcemia, hyperbilirubinemia, and polycythemia. As maternal euglycemia is obtained and maintained at optimal levels during pregnancy through medical nutrition therapy and other necessary interventions (see Chapters 6 and 7), the risk of complications is minimized and the maternal and fetal outcomes are improved.

REFERENCES

1. Sendag F, Terek MC, Itil IM, Oztekin K, Bilgin O. Maternal and perinatal outcomes in women with gestational diabetes mellitus as compared to nondiabetic controls. *J Reprod Med.* 2001;46:1057–1062.
2. Jensen DM, Sorensen B, Feilberg-Jorgensen N, Westergaard JG, Beck-Nielsen H. Maternal and perinatal outcomes in 143 Danish women with gestational diabetes mellitus and 143 controls with a similar risk profile. *Diabet Med.* 2000;17:281–286.
3. Jang HC, Cho NH, Min YK, Han IK, Jung KB, Metzger BE. Increased macrosomia and perinatal morbidity independent of maternal obesity and advanced age in Korean women with GDM. *Diabetes Care.* 1997;20:1582–1588.
4. Wood SL, Jick H, Sauve R. The risk of stillbirth in pregnancies before and after the onset of diabetes. *Diabet Med.* 2003;20:703–707.
5. National Heart Lung and Blood Institute. National High Blood Pressure Education Program: Working Group Report on High Blood Pressure in Pregnancy. Bethesda, Md: National Heart, Lung and Blood Institute (NHLBI); 2000. Available at: http://www.guideline.gov/summary/summary.aspx?doc_id=1478. Accessed December 7, 2004.
6. Sabai BM. Hypertension. In: Gabbe SG, Niebyl JR, Simpson JL. *Obstetrics: Normal and Problem Pregnancies.* 4th ed. Philadelphia, Pa: Churchill Livingstone; 2002:945–1004.
7. Barron WM. Hypertension. In: Barron WM, Lindheimer MD, eds. *Medical Disorders in Pregnancy.* St. Louis, Mo: Mosby; 2000.
8. Williams SR, Trahams CM. Management of pregnancy complications and special maternal disease conditions. In: Worthington-Roberts BS, Williams SR, eds. *Nutrition in Pregnancy and Lactation.* 6th ed. Madison, Wisc: Brown & Benchmark; 1997:254–291.
9. Hatton DC, McCarron DA. Dietary calcium and blood pressure in experimental models of hypertension. A review. *Hypertension.* 1994;23:513–530.
10. Villar J, Belizan JM, Fisher PJ. Epidemiologic observation on the relationship between calcium intake and preeclampsia. *Int J Gynaecol Obstet.* 1993;21:271–278.
11. Levine RJ, Hauth JC, Curet LB, Sibai BM, Catalano PM, Morris CD, DerSimonian R, Esterlitz JR, Raymond EG, Bild DE, Clemens JD, Cutler JA. Trial of calcium to prevent preeclampsia. *N Engl J Med.* 1997;337:69–76.

12. Lopez-Jaramillo P, Delgado F, Jacome P, Teran E, Ruano C, Rivera J. Calcium supplementation and the risk of preeclampsia in Ecuadorian pregnant teenagers. *Obstet Gynecol*. 1997;90:162–167.

13. Nordlander E, Hanson U, Persson B. Factors influencing neonatal morbidity in gestational diabetic pregnancy. *Br J Obstet Gynaecol*. 1989;96:671–678.

14. Garner PR, D'Alton ME, Dudley DK, Huard P, Hardie M. Preeclampsia in diabetic pregnancies. *Am J Obstet Gynecol*. 1990;163:505–508.

15. Berkowitz GS, Roman SH, Lapinski RH, Alvarez M. Maternal characteristics, neonatal outcome, and the time of diagnosis of gestational diabetes. *Am J Obstet Gynecol*. 1992;167:976–982.

16. Pettitt DJ, Knowler WC, Baird HR, Bennett PH. Gestational diabetes: infant and maternal complications of pregnancy in relation to third-trimester glucose tolerance in the Pima Indians. *Diabetes Care*. 1980;3:458–464.

17. Vambergue A, Nuttens MC, Goeusse P, Biausque S, Lepeut M, Fontaine P. Pregnancy-induced hypertension in women with gestational carbohydrate intolerance: the diagest study. *Eur J Obstet Gynecol Reprod Biol*. 2002;102:31–35.

18. Cousins L. Pregnancy complications among diabetic women: review 1965–1985. *Obstet Gynecol Surv*. 1987;42:140–149.

19. Jacobson JD, Cousins L. A population-based study of maternal and perinatal outcome in patients with gestational diabetes. *Am J Obstet Gynecol*. 1989;161:981–986.

20. Cohen HL. Polyhydramnios. In: Cohen HL, Sirit CJ, eds. *Fetal and Pediatric Ultrasound: A Casebook Approach*. New York, NY: McGraw Hill; 2001.

21. Uvena-Celebrezze J, Catalano PM. The infant of the woman with gestational diabetes mellitus. *Clin Obstet Gynecol*. 2000;43:127–139.

22. Hollingsworth DR. *Pregnancy, Diabetes and Birth: A Management Guide*. 2nd ed. Baltimore, Md: Williams and Wilkins; 1992.

23. Hedderson MM, Ferrara A, Sacks DA. Gestational diabetes mellitus and lesser degrees of pregnancy hyperglycemia: association with increased risk of spontaneous preterm birth. *Obstet Gynecol*. 2003;102:850–856.

24. Barrs VA. Obstetrical management. In: Hare JW, ed. *Diabetes Complicating Pregnancy: The Joslin Clinic Method*. New York, NY: Alan R Liss; 1989:99–124.

25. Xiong X, Saunders LD, Wang FL, Demianczuk NN. Gestational diabetes mellitus: prevalence, risk factors, maternal and infant outcomes. *Int J Gynaecol Obstet*. 2002;75:221–228.

26. Anoon SS, Rizk DE, Ezimokhai M. Obstetric outcome of excessively overgrown fetuses (≥5000 g): a case control study. *J Perinat Med*. 2003;31:295–301.

27. Conway DL. Delivery of the macrosomic infant: cesarean section versus vaginal delivery. *Semin Perinatol*. 2002;26:225–231.

28. Pettitt DJ, Baird HR, Aleck KA, Bennett PH, Knowler WC. Excessive obesity in offspring of Pima Indian women with diabetes during pregnancy. *N Engl J Med*. 1983;308:242–245.

29. Whitaker RC, Wright JA, Pepe MS, Seidel KD, Dietz WH. Predicting obesity in young adulthood from childhood and parental obesity. *N Engl J Med*. 1997;337:869–873.

30. Silverman BL, Rizzo TA, Cho NH, Metzger BE. Long-term effects of the intrauterine environment. *Diabetes Care*. 1998;21(Suppl 2):S142–S149.

31. Silverman BL, Rizzo T, Green OC, Cho NH, Winter RJ, Ogata ES, Richards GE, Metzger BE. Long-term prospective evaluation of offspring of diabetic mothers. *Diabetes*. 1991;40(Suppl 2):S121–S125.

32. Silverman BL, Ogata ES, Metzger BE. The offspring of the mother with diabetes. In: Porte D, Sherwin RS, eds. *Ellenberg and Rifkin's Diabetes Mellitus*. 5th ed. Stamford, Conn: Appleton and Lange; 1997:917–929.

33. Rizzo T, Metzger BE, Burns W, Burns K. Correlations between antepartum maternal metabolism and child intelligence. *N Engl J Med*. 1991;325:911–916.

34. Johar R, Rayburn W, Weir D, Eggert L. Birth weights in term infants. A 50-year perspective. *J Reprod Med*. 1988;33:813–816.

35. Sacks DA, Chen W. Estimating fetal weight in the management of macrosomia. *Obstet Gynecol Surv*. 2000;55:229–239.

36. American College of Obstetricians and Gynecologists. *Fetal Macrosomia*. Washington, DC: American College of Obstetricians and Gynecologists; 2000. ACOG Practice Bulletin Number 22.

37. Langer O. Fetal macrosomia: etiologic factors. *Clin Obstet Gynecol*. 2000;43:283–297.

38. Boulet SL, Alexander GR, Salihu HM, Pass MA. Macrosomic births in the United States: determinants, outcomes, and proposed grades of risk. *Am J Obstet Gynecol*. 2003;188:1372–1378.

39. Jimenez-Moleon JJ, Bueno-Cavanillas A, Luna-del-Castillo J, Garcia-Martin M, Lardelli-Claret P, Galvez-Vargas R. Impact of different levels of carbohydrate intolerance on neonatal outcomes classically associated with gestational diabetes mellitus. *Eur J Obstet Gynecol Reprod Biol*. 2002;102:36–41.

40. Persson B, Hanson U. Neonatal morbidities in gestational diabetes mellitus. *Diabetes Care*. 1998;21(Suppl 2):B79-B84.

41. Berkus MD, Conway D, Langer O. The large fetus. *Clin Obstet Gynecol*. 1999;42:766–784.

42. Kalkoff RK. Impact of maternal fuels and nutritional state on fetal growth. *Diabetes*. 1991; 40(Suppl 2):S61–S65.

43. Knopp RH, Bergelin RO, Wahl PW, Walden CE. Relationships of infant birth size to maternal lipoproteins, apoproteins, fuels, hormones, clinical chemistries, and body weight at 36 weeks gestation. *Diabetes*. 1985;34(Suppl 2):S71-S77.

44. Falluca F, Gargiulo P, Troili F, Zicari D, Pimpinella G, Maldonato A, Maggi E, Gerlini G, Pachi A. Amniotic fluid insulin, C peptide concentrations, and fetal morbidity in infants of diabetic mothers. *Am J Obstet Gynecol*. 1985;153:534–540.

45. Landon MB, Gabbe SG. Diabetes mellitus. In: Gabbe SG, Niebyl JR, Sampson JL, eds. *Obstetrics: Normal and Problem Pregnancies*. 4th ed. Philadelphia, Pa: Churchill Livingstone; 2002:1081–1116.

46. Thureen PJ, Deacon J, Hernandez JA, Hall DM. *Assessment and Care of the Well Newborn*. New York, NY: Elsevier Sanders; 2005.

47. Oh W. Neonatal outcome and care. In: Reece EA, Coustan DR, Gabbe SG, eds. *Diabetes in Women: Adolescence, Pregnancy, and Menopause*. Philadelphia, Pa: Lippincott, Williams & Wilkins; 2004:451–459.

48. Piper JM. Lung maturation in diabetes in pregnancy: if and when to test. *Sem Perinat*. 2002;26:206–209.

49. Langer O. A spectrum of glucose thresholds may effectively prevent complications in the pregnant diabetic patient. *Semin Perinatol*. 2002;26:196–205.

50. Kjos SL, Walther FJ, Montoro M, Paul RH, Diaz F, Stabler M. Prevalence and etiology of respiratory distress in infants of diabetic mothers: predictive value of fetal lung maturation tests. *Am J Obstet Gynecol*. 1990;163:898–903.

51. Landon MB, Gabe SG, Diabetes mellitus. In: Barron WM, Lindheimer MD. eds. *Medical Disorders in Pregnancy*. St. Louis, Mo: Mosby; 2000:71–100.

52. Cruikshank DP, Pitkin RM, Reynolds WA, Williams GA, Hargis GK. Altered maternal calcium homeostasis in diabetic pregnancy. *J Clin Endocrinol Metab*. 1980;50:264–267.

53. Widness JA, Cowett RM, Coustan DR, Carpenter MW, Oh W. Neonatal morbidities in infants of mothers with glucose intolerance in pregnancy. *Diabetes*. 1985;34(Suppl 2):S61–S65.

54. Moore TR, Diabetes in pregnancy. In: Creasy RK, Resnik R, Iams JD, eds. *Maternal-Fetal Medicine: Principles and Practice*. 5th ed. Philadelphia, Pa; 2004:1023–1061.

5

Maternal and Fetal Testing in Pregnancy

Alyce M. Thomas, RD

OBJECTIVES   After completing this chapter, you will be able to do the following:

1. Describe laboratory tests that are performed in cases of gestational diabetes mellitus (GDM).
2. Recognize the importance of self-monitoring in GDM.
3. List the tests used in fetal surveillance in GDM.
4. Explain the controversies of fetal testing to determine fetal well-being.

MATERNAL TESTING

During pregnancy, significant alterations occur in the maternal physiology. There is an expansion of plasma volume that results in a natural hemodilution of many blood components (1,2). Cardiac and pulmonary output, for example, is increased in pregnancy (1). Certain hormones, such as estrogen, progesterone, cortisol, human placental lactogen (hPL), and prolactin, are associated with decreased insulin sensitivity or insulin resistance (3). These changes are reflected in laboratory values that may differ from those of nonpregnant women.

In addition to the standard laboratory tests, such as the complete blood count (CBC) and urinalysis, the health care provider may order other tests for women with GDM. The tests performed include the creatinine clearance, A1C, and glycated serum protein (GSP).

Creatinine Clearance

Creatinine is produced from the degradation of creatine from the muscle mass (1,2). The clearance of creatinine from plasma to the kidneys is used to measure the glomerular filtration rate. In certain conditions, such as uncontrolled diabetes, however, creatinine may be reabsorbed. The creatinine clearance is increased in pregnancy because of the increased renal load. A decrease in the level could indicate impaired renal function. In this test, both blood and urine are collected.(1,2,4).

A1C

A1C (also known as glycosylated hemoglobin) measures the blood glucose level for an extended period of time (8 to 12 weeks) (5). The amount of glucose combined with the hemoglobin molecule reflects the degree of hyperglycemia. The value is expressed as a percentage of the total blood hemoglobin (1,2). A1C is also used as a predictor of the development of chronic complications associated with diabetes (5). The average life of the red blood cell is 120 days. The measure of the A1C will provide an indication of average blood glucose from the preceding 2 to 3 months (1,2). The correlation between A1C and mean plasma glucose levels can be found in Table 5.1 (6).

A1C testing helps the health care professional to determine the success in diabetes treatment and patient compliance. A1C is considered a better indicator of glycemic control than a single glucose measurement (1). It is not used to adjust insulin because it does not measure the blood glucose status at the time it was drawn. Nor is it used as a screening or diagnostic tool (1,4). Conditions, such as hemolytic anemia, could result in a false-negative report (7).

Although useful in the management of pregnancy with preexisting diabetes, the usefulness of A1C testing in GDM is unclear. It may prove useful if GDM is diagnosed before 20 weeks' gestation or to assess overall blood glucose control (8–10).

Glycated Serum Protein

GSP (fructosamine) provides a short-term measurement of glucose control. This test measures the serum glycosyl-protein formed by the reaction of glucose and protein molecules (9). Serum albumin has a short half-life of 14 to 20 days. GSP provides an index of glycemic

---

TABLE 5.1 Conversion of A1C to Mean Plasma Glucose Levels

A1C, %	Mean Blood Glucose, mg/dL
4	60
5	90
6	120
7	150
8	180
9	210
10	240
11	270
12	300
13	330

Source: Reprinted with permission from Diabetes Care and Education Dietetic Practice Group. *American Dietetic Association Guide to Diabetes Medical Nutrition Therapy and Education.* Chicago, Ill: American Dietetic Association; 2005.

statues from the preceding 1 to 2 weeks (5). It is useful in monitoring conditions in diabetes in which the A1C cannot be measured or the reliability is questionable (5). The role of GSP in pregnancy has not been established.

SELF-MONITORING

Blood Glucose

The monitoring of glycemic levels is an important component in the treatment of diabetes (11). However, the routine testing of blood glucose levels in GDM is controversial. There is no consensus about the frequency or necessity of blood glucose monitoring in GDM. Some professionals advocate self-monitoring in every woman with GDM; others argue that monitoring is necessary only in those treated with insulin (12,13). One reason for the lack of consensus is the paucity of information from large controlled trials. However, the Fourth International Workshop-Conference on Gestational Diabetes, the American Diabetes Association, and the American College of Obstetricians and Gynecologists (ACOG) agree that women with GDM should monitor their blood glucose levels (14–16). The frequency of glucose monitoring ranges from weekly in the office of a practitioner to daily self-monitoring (17). There is general agreement that monitoring using a reflectance glucose meter is far superior to the visual reagent strips (18).

Although the controversy continues, research has indicated that one of the most important reasons for glucose control is to decrease the risk of poor pregnancy outcome, including macrosomia. In its 2004 position statement on GDM, the American Diabetes Association concluded, "Daily self-monitoring of blood glucose appears to be superior to intermittent office monitoring of plasma glucose" (14). For the Association's target blood glucose levels in pregnancy, see Table 5.2 (14). The ACOG technical bulletin on GDM states that self-monitoring may be useful in decreasing potentially adverse outcomes, such as macrosomia (15).

If a woman consistently monitors her blood glucose and the levels are within the normal range, the frequency of testing could be decreased at the discretion of the health care provider (17). Dietetics professionals can use the results of monitoring to assess the effectiveness of the meal plan (19).

Test Accuracy

An important factor in self-monitoring is the accuracy of the test. Instructing the woman with GDM on the proper use of the glucose meter is the key to obtaining accurate results

TABLE 5.2 Target Plasma Blood Glucose in Pregnancy

Time	mg/dL*	mmol/L
Fasting	60–95	5.3
1 hour postprandial	<140	7.2
2 hour postprandial	<120	6.7

*To convert mg/dL to mmol/L, multiply by 0.0555.
Source: Reprinted with permission from American Diabetes Association. Gestational diabetes mellitus. Diabetes Care. 2004;27(Suppl 1):S88–S90.

(6). Instruction should address the amount of blood on the strip and care and maintenance of the glucose meter. The control solution is used to check the accuracy of the test strips. Health care providers must monitor the patient's technique at regular intervals. Laboratory tests should be conducted periodically to check the results from self-monitoring (5). If there are differences in excess of 10% between values from laboratory tests and self-monitored values, then self-monitoring testing procedures should be reevaluated (12). Glucose meters with memory capacity are preferred because they allow the independent verification of test results and help to avoid record-keeping errors (20).

Research has shown that in GDM, postprandial self-monitoring is associated with a lower incidence of complications (eg, fetal macrosomia, neonatal hypoglycemia, large-for-gestational-age infants, and cesarean section) than preprandial testing (15,21,22). In a study that compared preprandial and postprandial self-monitoring, Manderson and associates observed smaller triceps skinfold thickness in neonates when women monitored their glycemic levels after meals, which indicates a reduction in the incidence of fetal macrosomia (23). There appears to be no consensus as to whether 1- or 2-hour postprandial monitoring produces better outcomes. When comparing subjects who self-monitored blood glucose levels 1 hour after meals with those who self-monitored after 2 hours, Moses et al did not find differences in infant birth weight, percentage of women requiring insulin, or the total daily amount of insulin required (24). However, other studies found higher rates of abnormal values when women tested their blood glucose levels at 1 hour rather than at 2 hours postprandial (25–27).

Ketones

The role and benefits of urine ketone testing in pregnancy is controversial. In its 2004 position statement, the American Diabetes Association identified ketone testing as an important part in the monitoring of diabetes, including GDM (5).

The presence of ketonuria may indicate an inadequate intake of energy or carbohydrate (5,28). This starvation ketotic state may have a profound effect on fetal development. Research has suggested that ketonemia in the mother may decrease the intelligence in her children (29).

Ketones should be tested if a woman with GDM is experiencing nausea, is vomiting, or has sustained weight loss; if she is on a hypocaloric diet; or if she misses a meal (5,30). If the urine is positive for ketones, a blood test may confirm the presence of ketonemia. The frequency of testing may be daily in the morning at the beginning of the pregnancy, but it may decrease when blood glucose levels are stabilized and weight loss has stopped. Ketone monitoring is helpful in adjusting the energy and/or the carbohydrate content of the meal plan (19).

Blood ketone testing is preferred to urine ketone testing for diagnosing and monitoring for ketoacidosis (27). False-positive results can occur if the test strips are exposed to air for an extended period of time. Some glucose meters have the capacity to check blood ketone levels by testing for β-hydroxybutyric acid (27).

FETAL TESTING

Several tests have been developed to assess the well-being of the fetus. These tests include the nonstress test (NST), biophysical profile (BPP), ultrasound, the contraction stress test (CST), and amniocentesis. Although the practice of fetal surveillance in GDM is more common in women with other complications, such as hypertension or history of stillbirth, its use remains controversial because of the lack of well-designed studies (8,15,31,32). Women with GDM usually undergo more frequent testing than women with normal pregnancies. Because there is no consensus of opinion, the management criteria for testing may begin as early as 28 weeks' gestation or not until 36 weeks if there are no complications (17,15,33).

Nonstress Testing

The NST measures the acceleration of the fetal heart rate in response to fetal activity (34). The pregnant woman is seated in a reclining chair and the fetal heart rate is measured using a Doppler ultrasound. A test is reactive if there are at least two accelerations in the fetal heart rate in 20 minutes of monitoring. If there is no fetal movement during the time of NST, the test is considered nonreactive (34). This is not a cause for alarm; it may be an indication that the fetus is asleep. If this occurs, the woman may be instructed to eat or drink something to stimulate fetal movement. A nonreactive test for 40 minutes is an indication for further testing (8,34). The advantage of the NST is that it can be performed in the outpatient setting and can be completed in a relatively short time. In some centers, NSTs are performed as early as 36 weeks' gestation (8).

Contraction Stress Test

The CST measures fetal heart rate in response to uterine contractions. The test is usually conducted in the labor and delivery suite of a hospital (34). To induce mild contractions, a low dose of oxytocin is administered intravenously to the woman. Nipple stimulation may also be used to produce uterine contractions. Fetal heart rate is measured by Doppler ultrasound for 1 to 2 hours. The result of the test is either negative or positive. A negative test is associated with a good fetal outcome (34). A positive test may indicate fetal distress or intrauterine death (35).

Biophysical Profile

The biophysical profile (BPP) is a combination of an ultrasound with an NST (34,36). This test may be used in place of the contraction stress test. The BPP can evaluate the amniotic fluid volume and can detect major fetal abnormalities. There are five parameters studied: heart rate, breathing, body movement, muscle tone, and amniotic fluid volume.

Each parameter is given a score of either 0 or 2 points: a 2 is considered normal and 0 indicates an absence of the parameter. The highest score is 10, and the lowest is 0. A score of 10 indicates a normal fetus with a low risk of chronic asphyxia, whereas a score of 0 would indicate a strong suspicion of chronic asphyxia. If a BPP is indicated, it is performed once or twice weekly, beginning in the third trimester (34,36). For scoring guidelines, see Table 5.3 (31,34).

Ultrasonography

Ultrasonography is one of the most widely used methods of fetal testing (36,37). An ultrasound not only provides an image of the fetal anatomy; it can also estimate the date of conception by determining the gestational age through the use of several measurements (35,38). These parameters include abdominal circumference, fetal weight, femur length, and biparietal diameters (36). If there are discrepancies in any of the measurements, further evaluation may be necessary (33). Although the error rate may be as high as 15% to 20%, an ultrasound that predicts a fetal weight of more than 4,500 g could indicate the need for a cesarean delivery (31,36). Ultrasounds can also confirm multiple gestations and determine

TABLE 5.3 Scoring Guidelines for Biophysical Profile

Parameter	2 Points	0 Points
Heart rate	Presence ≥2 fetal heart accelerations of ≥15 beats/min and of at least 15 seconds duration associated with fetal movement in 30 min	<2 fetal heart accelerations or 1 acceleration of <15 beats/min in 30 min
Breathing	Presence of ≥30 seconds of fetal breathing movements in 30 min of observation	Absence of breathing or no episode of breathing for >30 seconds duration in 30 min
Body movement	At least 3 bodily or limb movements in 30 min of observation	≥2 episodes of bodily or limb movements in 30 min
Muscle tone	≥1 episode of motion of a limb from a position of flexion to extension and back to flexion	Slow extension with a return to partial flexion or movement of limb in full extension or absent fetal movement
Amniotic fluid volume	≥1 pocket of amniotic fluid that measures at least 2 cm in 2 perpendicular planes	No amniotic fluid pockets or a pocket <2 cm in 2 perpendicular planes

Source: Data are from references 32 and 35.

the location of the placenta and amniotic fluid, important factors in invasive procedures. A higher-resolution ultrasound can detect fetal abnormalities, such as nuchal folds, neural tube defects, and polydactyly (having more than the normal number of fingers and toes).

An ultrasound can detect fetal heartbeat and movement from early gestation. It is used in the third trimester to determine fetal presentation—whether vertex, breech, or transverse (37,38). Excessive or inadequate amniotic fluid associated with poor fetal outcome can be detected by ultrasound. Polyhydramnios, the excessive accumulation of amniotic fluid, is visible during the ultrasound (39). Anencephaly, hydrocephaly, and certain gastrointestinal malformations are associated with polyhydramnios and increase maternal blood glucose levels (40). Oligohydramnios, which can be detected by ultrasound, is a deficiency of amniotic fluid and is associated with renal anomalies, such as renal agenesis, or polycystic kidney disease (39).

Fetal Movement Counting

Fetal movement counting or kick counts is the pregnant woman's perception of fetal activity (10). This is a simple test that the woman can perform daily at home by counting the number of fetal movements within an allotted time during the third trimester (8). The woman is instructed to seek medical intervention if there is no perceived fetal activity during this time period.

Amniocentesis

Amniocentesis is an invasive test in which amniotic fluid is obtained for fetal cell analysis in a variety of genetic or chromosomal disorders (41,42). The test is performed by inserting a needle into the maternal abdomen. The needle placement is guided by the ultrasound, which locates a pocket of amniotic fluid and approximately 20 to 40 mL of fluid is extracted. Amniocentesis is usually performed at 15 to 20 weeks' gestation for chromosomal testing when sufficient fluid is present (42). Testing in the first trimester increases the risk of fetal loss (42). Although considered a relatively safe method of fetal analysis, amniocentesis is not without risks. The major complications associated with amniocentesis include the following (40,42):

- Infection
- Vaginal spotting
- Leakage of the amniotic fluid
- Maternal and/or fetal hemorrhage
- Premature rupture of the membranes
- Preterm labor
- Spontaneous abortion

If the fetus is at risk for fetal distress or respiratory distress syndrome, amniocentesis is also used in the third trimester of pregnancy to document lung maturity (8,42).

Maternal Serum Alpha Fetal Protein

Alpha fetal protein (AFP) is a glycoprotein found in the fetal serum by the third month of gestation (41). It is excreted by the fetal kidneys into the amniotic fluid and detected in the maternal serum around 14 to 18 weeks of pregnancy. A blood test for AFP is performed on the pregnant woman, and normal ranges are established for each week of gestation. These ranges are also called multiples of the median (MOMs). An elevated AFP (MOM = 2.0 to 2.5) may indicate that the fetus has a neural tube defect, such as spina bifida or anencephaly. A low level of AFP (MOM = 0.4) may indicate Down syndrome (41). Because AFP is a screening test, an amniocentesis may be used to confirm the AFP findings (8). Several factors may influence the AFP value, including miscalculation of the gestational age, maternal weight, multiple gestations, or fetal demise (42).

SUMMARY

The proliferation of maternal and fetal testing has resulted in earlier diagnosis of potentially harmful conditions, and, in certain cases, antenatal intervention. Noninvasive and invasive tests are performed to determine the well-being of the woman and fetus. In GDM, the higher risk for fetal morbidity or mortality may warrant increased monitoring, depending on the gestational age of the fetus and the glycemic levels of the pregnant woman. These tests include laboratory and self-testing of the urine or blood. Fetal testing includes ultrasound, stress tests, biophysical profiles, amniocentesis, and maternal alpha fetal protein sampling.

REFERENCES

1. Pagana KD, Pagana TJ. *Mosby's Manual of Diagnostic and Laboratory Tests.* 2nd ed. St. Louis, Mo: Mosby; 2000.
2. Sacher RA, McPherson RA. *Widmann's Clinical Interpretation of Laboratory Tests.* 11th ed. Philadelphia, Pa: FA Davis; 2000.
3. Yamashita H, Shao J, Friedman JE. Physiologic and molecular alterations in carbohydrate metabolism during pregnancy and gestational diabetes mellitus. *Clin Obstet Gynecol.* 2000;43:87–98.

4. Knudson PE, Weinstock RS, Henry JB. Carbohydrates. In: Henry JB, ed. *Clinical Diagnosis and Management by Laboratory Methods*. Philadelphia, Pa: WB Saunders; 2001:211–213.

5. Goldstein DE, Little RR, Lorenz RA, Malone JI, Nathan DM, Peterson CM; American Diabetes Association. Tests of glycemia in diabetes. *Diabetes Care*. 2004;27(Suppl 1):S91–S93.

6. Diabetes Care and Education Dietetic Practice Group. *American Dietetic Association Guide to Diabetes Medical Nutrition Therapy and Education*. Chicago, Ill: American Dietetic Association; 2005.

7. Sacks DB, Bruins DE, Goldstein DE, Maclaren NK, McDonald JM, Parrott M. Guidelines and recommendations for laboratory analysis in the diagnosis and management of diabetes mellitus. *Clin Chem*. 2002;48:436–472.

8. Jovanovic L, ed. *Medical Management of Pregnancy Complicated by Diabetes*. 3rd ed. Alexandria, Va: American Diabetes Association; 2000.

9. Rasouli N, Elbein SC. Management of diabetes mellitus. In: Reece EA, Coustan DR, Gabbe SG, eds. *Diabetes in Women; Adolescence, Pregnancy, and Menopause*. Philadelphia, Pa: Lippincott Williams and Wilkins; 2004:27–36.

10. Hollingsworth DR. Assessment of diabetic control during pregnancy. In: Hollingsworth DR, ed. *Pregnancy, Diabetes and Birth: A Management Guide*. Baltimore, Md: Williams and Wilkins; 1992.

11. Jovanovic L. Controversies in the diagnosis and treatment of gestational diabetes. *Cleve Clin J Med*. 2000;67:481–482, 485–486, 488.

12. Ryan EA, Nguyen G. Accuracy of glucose meter use in gestational diabetes. *Diabetes Technol Ther*. 2001;3:91–97.

13. Lehmann J. Screening, diagnosis and education of women with gestational diabetes. *Aust J Adv Nurs*. 1992;10:14–20.

14. American Diabetes Association. Gestational diabetes mellitus. *Diabetes Care*. 2004;27(suppl 1):S88–S90.

15. American College of Obstetricians and Gynecologists Committee on Practice Bulletins—Obstetrics. ACOG Practice Bulletin. Clinical management guidelines for obstetrician-gynecologists. Number 30, September 2001 (replaces Technical Bulletin Number 200, December 1994). Gestational diabetes. *Obstet Gynecol*. 2001;98:525–538.

16. Metzger BE, Coustan DR. Summary and recommendations of the Fourth International Workshop-Conference on Gestational Diabetes Mellitus. The Organizing Committee. *Diabetes Care*. 1998;21(Suppl 2):B161–B167.

17. Landon MB, Catalano PM, Gabbe SG. Diabetes mellitus. In: Gabbe SG, Niebyl JR, Simpson JL. *Obstetrics: Normal and Problem Pregnancies*. 4th ed. Philadelphia, Pa: Churchill Livingstone; 2002:1081–1116.

18. Kjos SL, Buchanan TA. Gestational diabetes mellitus. *N Engl J Med*. 1999;341:1749–1756.

19. American Dietetic Association. *Medical Nutrition Therapy Evidence-Based Guides for Practice: Nutrition Practice Guidelines for Gestational Diabetes Mellitus* [CD-ROM]. Chicago, Ill: American Dietetic Association; 2001.

20. Langer O. Maternal glycemic criteria for insulin therapy in gestational diabetes mellitus. *Diabetes Care*. 1998;21(Suppl 2):B91–B98.

21. deVeciana M, Major CA, Morgan MA, Asrat T, Toohey JS, Lien JM, Evans AT. Postprandial versus preprandial blood glucose monitoring in women with gestational diabetes mellitus. *N Engl J Med*. 1995;333:1237–1241.

22. Jovanovic L. American Diabetes Association's Fourth International Workshop-Conference on Gestational Diabetes Mellitus: summary and discussion. *Diabetes Care*. 1998;21(Suppl 2):B131–B137.

23. Manderson JG, Patterson CC, Hadden DR, Traub AI, Ennis C, McCance DR. Preprandial versus postprandial blood glucose monitoring in type 1 diabetic pregnancy: a randomized controlled clinical trial. *Am J Obstet Gynecol*. 2003;189:507–512.

24. Moses RG, Lucas EM, Knights S. Gestational diabetes mellitus. At what time should the postprandial glucose level be monitored? *Austral N Z J Obstet Gynaecol*. 1999;39:457–460.

25. Sivan E, Weisz B, Homko CJ, Reece EA, Schiff E. One or two hours postprandial glucose measurements: are they the same? *Am J Obstet Gynecol.* 2001;185:604–607.

26. Leguizamon G, Krupitzki H, Glujovsky D, Olivera Ravasi M, Reece EA. Blood glucose monitoring in gestational diabetes mellitus: 1- versus 2-h blood glucose determinations. *J Matern Fetal Neonatal Med.* 2002;12:384–388.

27. American Diabetes Association. Postprandial blood glucose. *Diabetes Care.* 2001;24:775–778.

28. Simon ER. Gestational diabetes mellitus: diagnosis, treatment, and beyond. *Diabetes Educ.* 2001;27:69–74.

29. Rizzo T, Metzger BE, Burns WJ, Burns K. Correlations between antepartum maternal metabolism and child intelligence. *N Engl J Med.* 1991;325:911–916.

30. Gabbe SG, Graves CR. Management of diabetes mellitus complicating pregnancy. *Obstet Gynecol.* 2003;102:857–868.

31. Farrell M. Improving the care of women with gestational diabetes. *MCN Am J Matern Child Nurs.* 2003;28:301–305.

32. Rosenn BM. Antenatal fetal testing in pregnancies complicated by gestational diabetes mellitus. *Semin Perinatol.* 2002;26:210–214.

33. Buchanan TA, Kjos SL, Schafer U, Peters RK, Xiang A, Byrne J, Berkowitz K, Montoro M. Utility of fetal measurements in the managements of gestational diabetes mellitus. *Diabetes Care.* 1998;21(Suppl 2):B99–B106.

34. Druzin ML, Gabbe SG, Reed KL. Antepartum fetal evaluation. In: Gabbe SG, Niebyl JR, Simpson JL. *Obstetrics: Normal and Problem Pregnancies.* 4th ed. Philadelphia, Pa: Churchill Livingstone; 2002:313–349.

35. Landon MB. Obstetric management of pregnancies complicated by diabetes mellitus. *Clin Obstet Gynecol.* 2000;43:65–74.

36. Vintzileos AM, Campbell WA, Rodis JF. Fetal biophysical profile. In: Winn HN, Hobbins JC. *Clinical Maternal-Fetal Medicine.* New York, NY: Parthenon Publishing Group; 2000:661–676.

37. Fleischer AC. *Sonography in Gynecology and Obstetrics: Just the Facts.* New York, NY: McGraw-Hill; 2004.

38. Chervenak FA, Gabbe SG. Obstetric ultrasound: assessment of fetal growth and anatomy. In: Gabbe SG, Niebyl JR, Simpson JL, eds. *Obstetrics: Normal and Problem Pregnancies.* Philadelphia, Pa: Churchill Livingstone; 2002:251–296.

39. Beattie RB. Disorders of amniotic fluid. In: Twining P, McHugo JM, Piling DW. *Textbook of Fetal Abnormalities.* London, England: Churchill Livingstone; 2000:75–88.

40. McManamon TG. Fetal monitoring. In: Davis BG, Mass D, Bishop M. *Principles of Clinical Laboratory Utilization and Consultation.* New York, NY: WB Saunders; 1999:319–324.

41. Jaffe R. Identification of fetal growth abnormalities in diabetes mellitus. *Semin Perinatol.* 2002;26:190–195.

42. Simpson JL. Genetic counseling and prenatal diagnosis. In: Gabbe SG, Niebyl JR, Simpson JL. *Obstetrics: Normal and Problem Pregnancies.* 4th ed. Philadelphia, Pa: Churchill Livingstone; 2002:187–219.

6

Medical Nutrition Therapy

Yolanda M. Gutierrez, MS, PhD, RD
Diane M. Reader, RD, CDE, consulting editor

OBJECTIVES   After completing this chapter, you will be able to do the following:

1. Describe the goals of the American Dietetic Association (ADA) medical nutrition therapy (MNT) evidence-based nutrition practice guidelines for gestational diabetes mellitus (GDM).
2. Explain the nutritional requirements of women during pregnancy.
3. Understand macronutrient requirements and their relationship to MNT in GDM.
4. Implement MNT for women with GDM.

MEDICAL NUTRITION THERAPY AND CLINICAL GOALS FOR GESTATIONAL DIABETES MELLITUS

In 1994, the ADA introduced the term "medical nutrition therapy" to describe the use of specific nutrition services to treat an illness, injury, or condition. MNT involves two phases: (*a*) assessment of the nutritional status of the client, and (*b*) treatment, which includes diet therapy, counseling, and the use of specialized nutrition supplements (1).

In 2001, ADA issued nutrition practice guidelines for GDM (2) and for type 1 and type 2 diabetes (3). The ideal/goal values listed in these guidelines are based on comprehensive reviews of published peer-reviewed research, as well as recommendations supported by national consensus committees.

According to the ADA nutrition practice guidelines for GDM, the clinical goals for the treatment of GDM are as follows (2):

1. To achieve and maintain normoglycemia
2. To consume adequate energy to promote appropriate gestational weight gain and avoid maternal ketosis
3. To consume food-providing nutrients necessary for maternal and fetal health

Registered dietitians assist women with GDM in achieving these outcomes by (*a*) assessing the individual's medical, social, and food history; (*b*) determining her unique clinical outcomes, such as the weight-gain goal; (*c*) developing a nutrition care plan; and (*d*) implementing and evaluating the care plan through multiple patient contacts.

ACHIEVING AND MAINTAINING NORMOGLYCEMIA

The first clinical outcome in the ADA nutrition practice guidelines for GDM (2) is unique to the management of GDM; the other two goals are shared by all pregnant women. In GDM, self-monitoring of blood glucose (SMBG), not A1C testing, is the primary test used to determine glucose control (see Chapter 5). Research demonstrates a direct relationship between postprandial blood glucose levels and rates of macrosomia, neonatal hypoglycemia, and cesarean delivery (4).

Controlling Carbohydrate Intake

Total Carbohydrate Intake

Carbohydrate is the primary nutrient affecting postprandial glucose levels, and in MNT for GDM the carbohydrate content of the food plan is modified to achieve and maintain normoglycemia. The ideal amount of carbohydrate for women with GDM is unknown, but carbohydrate intake is generally limited to about 40% to 45% of total daily energy intake (5–7). In a meal plan designed to control postprandial blood glucose values, carbohydrate intake is distributed throughout the day in three small- to moderate-sized meals and two to four snacks (2). Total daily carbohydrate intake should be individualized according to the woman's ability to tolerate carbohydrates, her unique eating pattern and food preferences, and her nutrition needs.

The established Dietary Reference Intake (DRI)/Recommended Dietary Allowance (RDA) for carbohydrate is 130 g/day for nonpregnant women and 175 g/day for pregnant or breastfeeding women (8). Forty percent of a 2,000-kcal/day food plan would provide 200 g carbohydrate, which is well above the minimum amount of carbohydrate needed to produce enough glucose for the brain to function (8,9).

Breakfast Carbohydrate Load

As a pregnancy progresses, hormone levels of human placental lactogen, progesterone, prolactin, and cortisol continuously increase. The increasing levels of these hormones cause changes in metabolism and alterations in the effectiveness of insulin to lower blood glucose levels (10,11). For most women with GDM, insulin resistance is greatest in the morning, because of the release of these hormones (10). Therefore, the breakfast carbohydrate load may need to be as low as 15 to 30 g (2). Specific nutrition and food recommendations should be determined and modified based on individual assessment and SMBG records. Adding foods that do not raise the postmeal glucose levels, such as proteins, can contribute calories and satisfy the woman's early morning hunger.

Amount of Carbohydrate vs Type of Carbohydrate

The total amount of carbohydrate has been shown to be a more important factor for glucose control than the source or type (12,13). Food records and postmeal monitoring of blood glucose can help identify foods that are less tolerated than others and can guide individual nutrition and food recommendations.

Research has shown that sucrose does not raise postmeal blood glucose levels any higher or faster than other carbohydrates (12). That stated, foods with sucrose, such as soda, pastries, desserts, and candy bars, are often high in total carbohydrate and contribute little to the nutritional value of a pregnant woman's diet. Generally, it is advised that women with GDM avoid these foods. However, if a woman does include sweet foods in her food plan, she should limit herself to a small portion, such as 15 g carbohydrate, which is substituted for another carbohydrate choice in her food plan (2,12).

Glycemic Index

The glycemic index (GI) was developed in the 1980s as a physiologic basis for classifying carbohydrates (14). It is a measure of the change in blood glucose after ingestion of carbohydrate-containing foods. Foods that rank low on the GI are digested and absorbed slowly and therefore produce gradual increases in blood glucose and insulin levels. Factors affecting the GI for particular foods include food form, ripeness, degree of processing, type of starch, cooking method, and fiber content. The first international tables of the GI were published in the *American Journal of Clinical Nutrition* in 1995 (15). The GI value of 100 is assigned to pure glucose, which is the reference food for all others (16). High-GI foods are ranked 70 or higher; low-GI foods have a GI less than 55. For a comparison of selected foods and the respective GI values, see Table 6.1 (16).

The GI may be useful to dietetics professionals working with women with GDM because it indicates foods that are likely to cause elevated postmeal glucose values. Highly processed breakfast cereals, instant potatoes, and instant noodles have high GIs (>70). Foods with a low GI (< 55) tend to be fresh, unprocessed, natural foods, such as milk, old-fashioned oatmeal, whole-grain breads, whole fruits, legumes (dried beans, peas, lentils), nuts, and pasta (16).

Diabetes professionals in Australia, Canada, and Europe have supported the GI as a tool for diabetes management for many years (17–19). The American Diabetes Association's position has been to emphasize the strong evidence for controlling the total amount of carbohydrate. Recently, the American Diabetes Association has identified the benefit of the use of the GI in this statement: "A recent analysis of the randomized controlled trials that have examined the efficacy of the glycemic index to overall blood glucose control indicates that the use of this technique can provide an additional benefit over that observed when total carbohydrate is considered alone" (13).

Insulin Therapy

If modification of the food plan alone does not provide the clinical outcome of achieving and maintaining normoglycemia, then insulin therapy is needed (2). Effective use of insulin requires that the woman eat consistent amounts of carbohydrate, so that the correct dose of insulin can be determined. Effective insulin use also requires the woman to eat at consistent time intervals. The use of insulin during pregnancy may allow for some flexibility in the amount of carbohydrate in a meal. For women using multiple daily injections or intensive forms of insulin therapy, insulin-to-carbohydrate ratios can be calculated to increase

TABLE 6.1 Selected Glycemic Index (GI) Values	
Food	*GI**
Apple, whole	38 ± 2
Apple juice, unsweetened	40 ± 1
Bagel, white	72
Bread, white	70 ± 0
Bread, whole wheat	71 ± 2
Banana, ripe, all yellow	51
Bran-type cereal, USA	38
Carrots, raw	47 ± 16
Corn, sweet, boiled	60
Cornflakes, USA	92
Kidney beans	28 ± 4
Long grain rice, parboiled	75 ± 7
Milk, nonfat	32 ± 5
Orange juice, reconstituted from frozen concentrate	57 ± 6
Peanuts	14 ± 8
Potatoes, instant mashed	97 ± 6
Potato, white, baked	85 ± 12
Sugar	68 ± 9
Soda pop—Coke	63
Snickers bar	68

*GI for glucose equals 100.
Source: Adapted from Foster-Powell K, Holt SH, Brand-Miller JC. International table of glycemic index and glycemic load values: 2002. *Am J Clin Nutr.* 2002;76:5–56. Adapted with permission by the *American Journal of Clinical Nutrition.* Copyright © 2002 Am J Clin Nutr. American Society for Clinical Nutrition.

flexibility in carbohydrate intake and to maintain the tight glycemic control needed during pregnancy. Prevention and treatment of hypoglycemia is an important topic to discuss with women on insulin therapy (see Chapter 7).

ADEQUATE ENERGY CONSUMPTION

The second clinical outcome for management of GDM, consuming adequate energy to provide appropriate gestational weight gain and avoid maternal ketosis, is important for two reasons. First, research supports appropriate weight gain, based on body mass index (BMI), as critical for normal fetal development in all pregnant women (9). Second, as women with GDM begin to modify their food intake to control postprandial glucose values, they are at risk of undereating, weight loss, and increased ketosis.

Weight-Gain Goals

Optimal neonatal outcomes occur in women who gain the recommended weight based on the Institute of Medicine guidelines for prepregnancy BMI (9). Therefore, weight-gain goals are based on the woman's prepregnancy BMI (see Table 6.2) (20). For weight-gain ranges based on weight categories and BMI, see Table 6.3 (9,21).

Women with GDM, particularly those who are overweight or obese, benefit from nutrition counseling, to monitor the rate of weight gain during pregnancy. A dietetics professional supported by a team of health care providers should individually evaluate each case and provide the necessary education to achieve weight-gain goals.

It is not unusual for women with GDM to experience some weight loss after beginning their nutrition plan. The weight loss may be attributed to changes in the amount of carbohydrate and total energy consumed; also women with GDM may find nutrient-dense foods more filling and consequently eat smaller amounts of high-calorie/high-fat foods. Evaluating daily food records is a way to determine whether women are consuming adequate calories or whether they are undereating to control glucose values.

Energy Needs in Pregnancy

The energy cost for a full-term pregnancy in which the woman gains 12.5 kg (27.5 lb) and delivers a 3.3-kg (7.33-lb) baby is estimated to be 80,000 kcal (8,22). Unless a woman is underweight, energy intake does not need to increase in the first trimester. Energy requirements increase during the second and third trimesters, but there is great variability in the average change in energy needs between women.

Formulas stating x number of kilocalories per kilogram body weight have not been published for pregnant women. According to the Institute of Medicine, "Nonpregnant prediction equations based on weight are not accurate during pregnancy, since metabolic rate increases disproportionately to the increase in weight" (9). In view of the complexities and variability of the daily human diet, energy recommendations should *not* be based on a woman's actual food intake.

Historically, dietitians have recommended adding about 300 kcal/day to a woman's prepregnancy energy needs (calculated using a formula such as the Harris Benedict equation) (22,23). For example, if a normal-weight, nonpregnant American woman ingests about 2,200 kcal/day, then her average intake during the second and third trimesters should be about 2,500 kcal/day (8,22). Energy demands are thought to be the greatest between 10 and 30 weeks' gestation.

The Institute of Medicine has recently released new research-based energy intake calculations for pregnancy. These indicate that energy needs during pregnancy are higher than previously thought. To calculate a pregnant woman's energy needs using the Institute of Medicine's formulas, the clinician must first calculate the estimated energy requirement (EER) (note: EER is not used for overweight individuals). The equation for calculating the EER for women 19 years and older (8) is as follows:

$$EER = 354 - (6.91 \times A) + PA \times (9.36 \times Wt + 726 \times Ht)$$

Where: A = age (years); PA = physical activity coefficient; Wt = weight (kg); Ht = height (meters).

There are four physical activity coefficients, one for each of the four physical activity levels (PALs) (see Table 6.4) (8,22). PAL is defined as the ratio of total energy expenditure to basal energy expenditure (8).

TABLE 6.2 Body Mass Index (BMI)

Height, in \ BMI	Normal						Overweight					Obese										Extreme Obesity															
	19	20	21	22	23	24	25	26	27	28	29	30	31	32	33	34	35	36	37	38	39	40	41	42	43	44	45	46	47	48	49	50	51	52	53	54
																		Body weight, lb																		
58	91	96	100	105	110	115	119	124	129	134	138	143	148	153	158	162	167	172	177	181	186	191	196	201	205	210	215	220	224	229	234	239	244	248	253	258
59	94	99	104	109	114	119	124	128	133	138	143	148	153	158	163	168	173	178	183	188	193	198	203	208	212	217	222	227	232	237	242	247	252	257	262	267
60	97	102	107	112	118	123	128	133	138	143	148	153	158	163	168	174	179	184	189	194	199	204	209	215	220	225	230	235	240	245	250	255	261	266	271	276
61	100	106	111	116	122	127	132	137	143	148	153	158	164	169	174	180	185	190	195	201	206	211	217	222	227	232	238	243	248	254	259	264	269	275	280	285
62	104	109	115	120	126	131	136	142	147	153	158	164	169	175	180	186	191	196	202	207	213	218	224	229	235	240	246	251	256	262	267	273	278	284	289	295
63	107	113	118	124	130	135	141	146	152	158	163	169	175	180	186	191	197	203	208	214	220	225	231	237	242	248	254	259	265	270	278	282	287	293	299	304
64	110	116	122	128	134	140	145	151	157	163	169	174	180	186	192	197	204	209	215	221	227	232	238	244	250	256	262	267	273	279	285	291	296	302	308	314
65	114	120	126	132	138	144	150	156	162	168	174	180	186	192	198	204	210	216	222	228	234	240	246	252	258	264	270	276	282	288	294	300	306	312	318	324
66	118	124	130	136	142	148	155	161	167	173	179	186	192	198	204	210	216	223	229	235	241	247	253	260	266	272	278	284	291	297	303	309	315	322	328	334
67	121	127	134	140	146	153	159	166	172	178	185	191	198	204	211	217	223	230	236	242	249	255	261	268	274	280	287	293	299	306	312	319	325	331	338	344
68	125	131	138	144	151	158	164	171	177	184	190	197	203	210	216	223	230	236	243	249	256	262	269	276	282	289	295	302	308	315	322	328	335	341	348	354
69	128	135	142	149	155	162	169	176	182	189	196	203	209	216	223	230	236	243	250	257	263	270	277	284	291	297	304	311	318	324	331	338	345	351	358	365
70	132	139	146	153	160	167	174	181	188	195	202	209	216	222	229	236	243	250	257	264	271	278	285	292	299	306	313	320	327	334	341	348	355	362	369	376
71	136	143	150	157	165	172	179	186	193	200	208	215	222	229	236	243	250	257	265	272	279	286	293	301	308	315	322	329	338	343	351	358	365	372	379	386
72	140	147	154	162	169	177	184	191	199	206	213	221	228	235	242	250	258	265	272	279	287	294	302	309	316	324	331	338	346	353	361	368	375	383	390	397
73	144	151	159	166	174	182	189	197	204	212	219	227	235	242	250	257	265	272	280	288	295	302	310	318	325	333	340	348	355	363	371	378	386	393	401	408
74	148	155	163	171	179	186	194	202	210	218	225	233	241	249	256	264	272	280	287	295	303	311	319	326	334	342	350	358	365	373	381	389	396	404	412	420
75	152	160	168	176	184	192	200	208	216	224	232	240	248	256	264	272	279	287	295	303	311	319	327	335	343	351	359	367	375	383	391	399	407	415	423	431
76	156	164	172	180	189	197	205	213	221	230	238	246	254	263	271	279	287	295	304	312	320	328	336	344	353	361	369	377	385	394	402	410	418	426	435	443

Source: National Heart, Lung, and Blood Institute. Body mass index table. Available at: http://www.nhlbi.nih.gov/guidelines/obesity/bmi_tbl.htm. Accessed March 17, 2005.

TABLE 6.3   Recommended Weight Gain for Pregnant Women

Category	Prepregnancy BMI*	Recommended Total Weight Gain, lb
Underweight	<18.5	28–40
Normal weight	18.5–24.9	25–35
Overweight	25–29.9	15–25
Obesity (Class 1)	30–34.9	≥15
Obesity (Class 2)	35–39.9	Not available
Obesity (Class 3)	≥40	Not available

*Young adolescents, African-American women, and smokers should strive for gains at the upper end of the recommended ranges. These women tend to give birth to smaller infants. Women shorter than 62 inches should strive for gains at the lower end of the ranges.
Source: Data are from references 9 and 21.

TABLE 6.4   Physical Activity Coefficients for Adult Women

PAL*	PA
Sedentary: ≥1.0 < 1.4	1.0
Low active: ≥1.4 < 1.6	1.12
Active: ≥1.6 < 1.9	1.27
Very active: ≥1.9 < 2.5	1.45

Abbreviations: PA, physical activity coefficient; PAL, physical activity level.
*PAL is defined as the ratio of total energy expenditure to basal energy expenditure.
Source: Data are from references 8 and 22.

The formulas for estimating the energy requirements for pregnant women who have normal weight are as follows (8):

- 1st trimester = Adult EER + 0
- 2nd trimester = Adult EER + 160 kcal (8 kcal/wk × 20 wk) + 180 kcal
- 3rd trimester = Adult EER + 272 kcal (8 kcal/wk × 34 wk) + 180 kcal

The fetus appears to use about 160 and 272 kcal/day in the second and third trimesters, respectively. The woman's basal energy needs increase by about 180 kcal/day in the second and third trimesters.

In women with GDM who are managed in an outpatient setting, energy needs are usually evaluated indirectly by monitoring the woman's physical activity, appetite, food intake, blood glucose levels, ketone records, and weight change. Most clinicians do not calculate energy needs unless the woman is experiencing problems with excessive weight loss or weight gain. In those situations, a formula will guide the dietitian to develop a food plan in the appropriate calorie range.

Energy Needs and Overweight or Obesity

As noted earlier in this chapter, the EER formulas are not used for overweight or obese individuals. Historically, an adjusted body weight has been used with the Harris-Benedict formula to determine energy needs for nonpregnant obese women (22,24):

$$(ABW - IDBW) \times 0.25 + IDBW = \text{Weight to be used for calculating energy needs}$$

Where: ABW = actual body weight (kg); IDBW = ideal desirable body weight (kg); 0.25 = percentage of excess body weight that is metabolically active.

The Institute of Medicine report on energy needs for pregnancy was limited to normal BMI (18.5–24.0). At this time, there is no formula supported by research to determine the energy needs in overweight or obese pregnant women. Clinicians are encouraged to monitor weight gain regularly in these women and to advise them individually to adjust intake of calories, fats, and carbohydrates, to keep weight gain to about 0.5 lb/week (9).

CONSUMING FOOD-PROVIDING NUTRIENTS NECESSARY FOR MATERNAL AND FETAL HEALTH

Consuming foods that provide nutrients necessary for maternal and fetal health (the third clinical outcome for MNT in GDM) is a goal for all pregnant women, including those with GDM. An adequate supply of nutrients is probably the single most important environmental factor affecting pregnancy outcome. For a comparison of daily nutrient requirements for nonpregnant and pregnant women, see Table 6.5 (8,22,25–28).

It is critical that women with GDM not exclude healthful carbohydrate foods, such as fruit and milk, in an effort to improve glucose control. A common strategy to achieve the simultaneous goal of glucose control and good nutrition is to move fruit and milk servings to snack time and to keep starch carbohydrates at meal time. Avoiding fruit or juice at breakfast may improve postbreakfast glycemic control.

Fresh vegetables, especially broccoli, spinach, and greens, should be eaten in liberal amounts. Milk (nonfat, low-fat, reduced-fat, or whole) is recommended; the type used depends on the woman's individual energy needs.

Dietetics professionals should note that the dietary principles for singleton pregnancy can be followed for women with multiple gestations who develop GDM, if adjustments are made to energy and nutrient levels according to the weight-gain requirements.

Protein

Protein needs increase during the second and third trimesters by 25 g/day (8). The RDA for protein in nonpregnant women is about 46 g/day (8) or 0.8 g protein/kg/day. For example, the RDA for protein for a nonpregnant woman who weighs 64 kg (140 lb) is 51 g/day (64 × 0.8 = 51). If this woman becomes pregnant, the RDA for protein increases by 25 g from the second trimester to term, to 76 g/day (51 g + 25 g = 76 g/day). This 25 g of additional protein is equivalent to 1.1 g protein per kg desirable body weight (8).

Maternal protein synthesis increases to support expansion of the blood volume, uterus, and breasts. Fetal and placental proteins are synthesized by amino acids supplied by the woman. The 2002 DRI report for macronutrients (8) determined that Tolerable Upper Intake Levels for protein and individual amino acids could not be set at that time, because the data were conflicting or inadequate. However, it was noted that caution is warranted in consuming protein levels significantly above those normally found in foods.

TABLE 6.5 Daily Nutrient Requirements During Pregnancy

Nutrient (References)	Nonpregnant Women, Age 15–50 y	Pregnant Women
Energy, kcal (8,22)	2200	+300 (2nd and 3rd trimesters)
Protein, g (8)	46	+25
Vitamin A, µg RAE (25)	700	Age 14–18 y: 750
		Age 19–50 y: 770
Vitamin D, µg (26)	5	5
Vitamin K, µg (25)	90	Age 14–18 y: 75
		Age 19–50 y: 90
Vitamin C, mg (27)	75	Age 14–18 y: 80
		Age 19–50 y: 85
Thiamin, mg (28)	1.1	1.4
Riboflavin, mg (28)	1.1	1.4
Niacin, mg NE (28)	14	18
Vitamin B-6, mg (28)	1.3	1.9
Folate, µg FE (28)	400	600
Vitamin B-12, µg (28)	2.4	2.6
Calcium, mg (26)	1000	Age 14–18 y: 1300
		Age 19–50 y: 1000
Phosphorus, mg (26)	700	Age 14–18 y: 1250
		Age 19–50 y: 700
Magnesium, mg (26)	360–265	Age 14–18 y: 400
		Age 19–50 y: 360
Iron, mg (25)	18	27
Zinc, mg (25)	8	Age 14–18 y: 12
		Age 19–50 y: 11
Iodine, µg (25)	150	220
Selenium, µg (27)	55	60

Protein intake in GDM may be slightly higher than the recommended DRI levels, because the amount of carbohydrate in the diet is decreased (2).

Dietary Fat

With regard to dietary fat intake levels, there are two main factors to consider: the fat's impact on body weight and the individual's plasma lipoprotein profiles. If a woman is overweight or gaining weight at a higher rate than is recommended, a reduction in total fat may be warranted, to induce a lower total energy intake. With regard to the type of fat, women with GDM should be advised to minimize intake of saturated and *trans* fatty acids and to limit foods high in cholesterol while consuming a nutritionally adequate diet.

Current evidence on dietary fat quality suggests that saturated fatty acids tend to increase low-density lipoprotein (LDL) cholesterol levels, whereas monounsaturated and polyunsaturated fatty acids tend to decrease LDL cholesterol levels (29). The n-3 fatty acids—eicosapentaenoic acid (EPA) (20:5n-3) and docosahexaenoic acid (DHA) (22:6n-3)—are associated with decreased triglyceride levels in patients with dyslipidemia and a decreased risk of developing coronary heart disease (CHD) (29). Dietary *trans* fatty acids are associated with increased LDL cholesterol levels (29).

A nutrient-rich diet for pregnancy should include n-3 and n-6 fatty acids. N-3 fatty acids, also called linolenic acid, can be found in all fish and seafood, egg yolks, the leaves and seeds of many plants, soybeans, nuts, and oils such as canola, flaxseed, olive, and walnut. N-6 fatty acids, also called linoleic acid, can be found in nuts, including walnuts, peanuts, almonds; seeds, such as sunflower seeds; and oils, such as corn, safflower, sunflower, and soybean.

Folate

Folate is involved in cell multiplication and DNA synthesis. The requirement for folate in a pregnancy is 600 µg/day (see Table 6.6) (28). Women with multiple gestations, mothers nursing more than one infant, chronic or heavy alcohol users, and women on chronic anticonvulsant or methotrexate therapy may need intakes higher than the RDA.

Folate supplementation is associated with a decreased incidence of small-for-date births and neural tube defects (30). Since 1998, when folic acid fortification of cereal grains began, intake in women has increased from 80 to 100 µg/day (28).

A deficiency of folate in pregnancy may result in an increased risk for birth defects, such as neural tube defects or Down syndrome, preterm delivery, and elevated serum homocysteine levels, which may be a predictor of poor pregnancy outcomes (28). In a study to determine the effect of plasma homocysteine on pregnancy outcomes, Vollset et al (31) compared the upper to lower quartiles of plasma homocysteine levels of 14,492 pregnancies in 5,883 Norwegian women. The results showed a higher risk of poor pregnancy outcome in the women with increased homocysteine levels: 203% higher risk of stillbirth; 101% higher risk of very-low-birth-weight infants; 32% higher risk of preeclampsia; 38% higher risk of preterm delivery; 313% higher risk of placental abruption; and increased risk of clubfoot and neural tube defects (31).

Other important points to consider in folate recommendations are the following:

- All women of reproductive age who are capable of becoming pregnant should take 400 µg additional folate from food or supplements (28).
- Supplementation begun in later pregnancy may still provide benefit.

TABLE 6.6   Daily Folate Recommendations* for Women, Age 14 to 50 Years

	EAR, µg[†]	RDA, µg[‡]	UL, µg[§]
Nonpregnant		400	
Pregnant (singleton)	520	600	Age 14–18 y: 800
			Age 19 + y: 1000

Abbreviations: EAR, estimated average requirement; RDA, recommended dietary allowance; UL, Tolerable Upper Intake Level

*Dietary Folate Equivalents.

[†]Recommendation meets the needs for 50% of the population.

[‡]Recommendation meets the needs for 97.5% of the population.

[§]Highest average daily intake likely to pose no risk of adverse health effects.

Source: Data are from reference 28.

- One microgram of food folate or 1 dietary folate equivalent (DFE) equals 0.6 µg synthetic folate.
- Women at risk of vitamin B-12 deficiency, such as vegans, may be at increased risk of the precipitation of neurologic disorders if excessive folate is consumed (28).

Calcium

Peak bone mass attained by the third decade of life is an important determinant of osteoporosis risk (32,33). Approximately 60% to 80% of the variance is attributed to genetics, leaving modifiable factors, such as diet and physical activity, to influence the attainment of a person's genetic programmed peak bone mass (34,35). The DRI for calcium in pregnancy is 1,300 mg for ages 14 to 18 and 1,000 mg for ages 19 to 50 (26).

The Institute of Medicine's recommendations for pregnancy are based on the assumption that most of the peak bone mass is attained by 18 years of age. Because of increased efficiency of calcium absorption, the requirements during pregnancy are similar to those in the nonpregnant state. Studies document no significant increase in calcium absorption during lactation (26,36).

Iron

The "iron cost" of a full-term pregnancy has been calculated to be about 1,000 mg (9). This translates to a requirement for absorbed iron of approximately 3 mg/day during pregnancy. In the nonpregnant state, iron absorption from food is only about 10%. The amount of iron absorbed from food during pregnancy increases to 25% from the beginning of the second trimester. The Institute of Medicine recommends an iron supplement of 30 mg ferrous iron in the second and third trimesters (9). The average American's diet contains only about 6 mg iron/1,000 kcal (9).

Nutrient Adequacy in Closely Spaced Pregnancies

Women with closely spaced pregnancies are at increased risk of entering the reproductive cycle with reduced reserves. Maternal nutrient depletion may contribute to an increased incidence of preterm births and fetal growth retardation as well as an increased risk of maternal mortality and morbidity (37). For example, marginal intakes of iron and folic acid during the reproductive period induce a poor maternal status for these nutrients during the interconception interval. Poor iron and folic acid status have been associated with preterm births and fetal growth retardation (37). Supplementation with food and micronutrients during the interconception period may improve pregnancy outcomes and maternal health in women (37,38).

VEGETARIANISM AND PLANT-BASED DIETS

There are three main categories of vegetarian diets: (*a*) lacto-vegetarian, which includes dairy products; (*b*) lacto-ovo-vegetarian, which includes dairy products and eggs; and (*c*) vegan, which excludes all foods of animal origin. Other types of plant-based diets include macrobiotic, which consists of grains, legumes, and vegetables; and fruitarian, a diet based primarily on fruit.

In a joint position statement by the American Dietetic Association and the Dietitians of Canada, appropriately planned vegetarian diets were found to be "healthful, nutritionally adequate, and provide health benefits in the prevention of certain diseases" (39). In the United States, approximately 2.5% of the population, or nearly 5 million people, are vegetarians (39). Their diets tend to be lower in fats and cholesterol, but higher in fiber and magnesium, than other diets. The intake of certain vitamins and minerals may be lower in vegans. In particular, vitamin D, calcium, and zinc are of special concern, because food sources for these nutrients are primarily animal based.

Vegetarian women can promote healthy pregnancies by following the DRIs. Studies have shown that women can meet their daily requirements with a vegetarian diet (39,40). The birth weights of infants whose mothers are vegetarian are no different from those whose mothers are nonvegetarian (41). The weight-gain recommendations for pregnant women with a normal BMI are the same for vegetarians and nonvegetarians (25 to 35 lb).

For vegetarians with GDM, the basis of the diet plan is similar to that for nonvegetarian women with GDM: lower amounts of carbohydrate (40%–45% of energy intake), moderate protein (15%–20%), and the remaining calories as fat (30%–40%). Carbohydrate intake should be limited to 15 to 30 g at breakfast, to control glucose levels during early morning insulin resistance. Choosing foods with whole grains and those that cause a lower glycemic response may help to avoid postprandial glycemic excursions (42).

Protein sources for lacto-ovo vegetarians include eggs and dairy products. Legumes, nuts, seeds, tofu, tempeh, textured vegetable protein, and fortified soy milk are protein sources used by vegans.

Vegetarians tend to have adequate total fat intakes, but their diets may be low in the n-3 fatty acids DHA and EPA, fats that are typically found in fish and eggs. Vegetarian foods high in n-3 fatty acids, such as flaxseed or flaxseed oil, canola oil, or English walnuts, need to be incorporated into the diet, or the individual may take a vegetarian DHA supplement from microalgae (39). The intake of foods containing n-6 fatty acids should be limited because of their interference with n-3 fatty acid production.

Vitamin B-12 is necessary in amino acid and fatty acid metabolism, and in the prevention of megaloblastic anemia. An inadequate maternal intake of vitamin B-12 in pregnancy may put the fetus at risk for deficiency. The best food source of vitamin B-12 is animal products. Vegans can meet their requirements with foods fortified with vitamin B-12 or a vitamin B-12 supplement (43). Folic acid intakes in vegetarian women tend to be higher than in nonvegetarian women (39); however, folate supplementation may be necessary to meet the recommendation of 600 µg in pregnancy.

Vegans tend to consume less calcium than nonvegans, and a supplement is necessary if nondairy food sources of calcium (dark-green leafy vegetables, calcium-fortified orange juice, or calcium-fortified soy milk) are not consumed at amounts to meet the daily requirements (39). Adequate levels of vitamin D are necessary for calcium absorption. Vitamin D is derived primarily from animal sources or sunlight. Most women cannot depend on sufficient sun exposure to meet their vitamin D requirements, so vegetarian women may need to use a vitamin D supplement or consume foods fortified with vitamin D.

Both vegetarian and nonvegetarian pregnant women are at increased risk of iron deficiency (39,43). Heme iron is derived from animal sources and is more bioavailable than nonheme iron. Factors affecting the absorption of nonheme iron sources include phytates and tannins. Iron supplementation is routinely recommended in pregnancy for all women. Zinc is necessary in DNA synthesis and a zinc deficiency in pregnancy may be associated with congenital anomalies or fetal death (9). Phytates interfere with zinc absorption, and higher intakes of zinc may be necessary for vegetarian women, although no extra supplementation is recommended (43).

USE OF CAFFEINE AND NONNUTRITIVE SWEETENERS IN PREGNANCY

Caffeine

Caffeine is a naturally occurring product that can affect the central nervous system within 15 minutes of its ingestion. The effects are slight increases in blood pressure and heart rate. No studies have linked caffeine consumption to birth defects in humans, although caffeine is known to cross the placenta and can affect fetal heart rate and breathing (38,44,45).

Caffeine has been linked to an increase in first trimester spontaneous abortions in women who consumed more than 300 mg/day (38). There is some limited evidence that suggests that moderate to heavy caffeine use may lower infant birth weight, increase the risk of preterm labor, and delay conception (38,46). During pregnancy, caffeine intake should be limited to less than 300 mg/day (38).

Nonnutritive Sweeteners

Nonnutritive sweeteners have a sweet taste but do not provide energy. The Food and Drug Administration (FDA) has approved five nonnutritive sweeteners: saccharin, aspartame, acesulfame potassium (acesulfame K), sucralose, and, most recently, neotame. The effects of nonnutritive sweeteners on the reproductive abilities in females and males and on the developing fetus have been studied extensively (38,47,48).

Of the five approved nonnutritive sweeteners, concerns have been raised about the use of saccharin and aspartame during pregnancy. Saccharin is known to cross the placenta and may remain in the fetal tissues because of low fetal clearance (47). Although animal studies have suggested a possible bladder cancer risk in neonatal exposure to saccharin, no risk has been found in human subjects (48). Because saccharin was removed from the list of potential carcinogens, its use in pregnancy is considered safe (49).

Aspartame is a dipeptide that is hydrolyzed to aspartic acid, phenylalanine, and methanol. While amino acids cross the placenta, the use of aspartame within the FDA guidelines appears to be safe in pregnancy. In animals, an aspartame load does not change fetal exposure to aspartic acid (38,49). Women who have phenylketonuria (PKU) should restrict their intake of aspartame.

Aspartame does not cross into breastmilk (38,49). Saccharin and acesulfame-K do cross into breastmilk; however, the effect on the infant is unknown.

In summary, nonnutritive sweeteners approved by the FDA are considered safe for use during pregnancy when they are used within the Acceptable Daily Intakes. As a general guideline, three to four servings or portions per day are conservative limits for use. Nonnutritive sweeteners not approved for use in the United States include alitame, cyclamates, neohesperidine, stevia, and thaumatin (38,49).

IMPLEMENTING MNT

The process of MNT begins with the confirmed diagnosis of GDM. The primary care provider refers the patient to a registered dietitian to receive MNT for GDM. MNT includes assessment, diagnosis, intervention, and monitoring and evaluation of clinical outcomes (see Figure 6.1) (2).

Initial Session

For the initial session, registered dietitians should have the following materials (2):

Nutrition Practice Guidelines for GDM

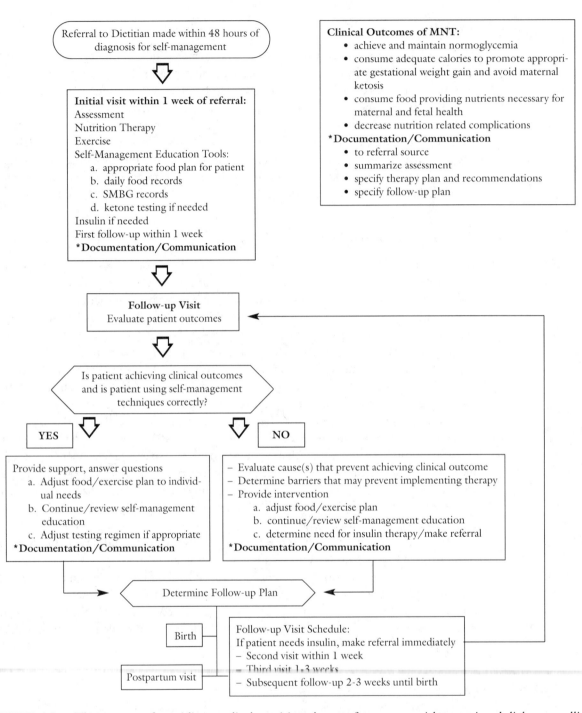

FIGURE 6.1. The process of providing medical nutrition therapy for women with gestational diabetes mellitus. Adapted with permission from American Dietetic Association. *Medical Nutrition Therapy Evidence-Based Guides for Practice: Nutrition Practice Guidelines for Gestational Diabetes Mellitus* [CD-ROM]. Chicago, Ill: American Dietetic Association; 2001.

- Signed referral form from provider (Appendix A, Figure A.1)
- Nutrition questionnaire (Appendix A, Figure A.2) or other history form
- 24-hour recall or food record (Appendix A, Figure A.3) and, if possible, food frequency questionnaire (Appendix A, Figure A.4)
- Nutrition assessment form and care plan (Appendix A, Figure A.5) and food plan calculation form (Appendix A, Figure A.6)
- Prenatal weight-gain grid (Figures 6.2 and 6.3) (50)
- Nutrition education materials, such as *Basic Carbohydrate Counting* (51), *My Food Plan for Gestational Diabetes* (52), or *Gestational Diabetes: Caring for Yourself and Your Baby* (53)
- Gestational diabetes blood glucose and food record form (Appendix A, Figure A.7) or another form to record both food intake and blood glucose results
- Additional printed educational materials as necessary (eg, on the use of nutritive and nonnutritive sweeteners, calcium sources, and fish consumption during pregnancy)
- Educational tools, such as food models, product samples, measuring utensils, etc.
- Billing form
- Progress note or system-appropriate documentation form

Ideally, the initial session lasts approximately 60 minutes. During this time, the registered dietitian should complete the nutrition assessment using pertinent physical, maternal, and laboratory data, usual dietary intake, eating schedule, and food preferences. Clinical outcomes for the woman, including a weight-gain goal and an estimation of the woman's energy or carbohydrate requirements, should be determined. Using data from the nutrition assessment, the registered dietitian can develop an appropriate food plan to implement MNT. After developing the food plan, the dietitian uses a patient education tool to teach the client about it. The tool should be appropriate for the client's educational and cultural background.

The registered dietitian should review prenatal weight gain with the woman and discuss weight-gain goals. The role of exercise in good health should be explained, and regular, consistent exercise should be encouraged within medically appropriate parameters. The client should be instructed regarding record keeping, and a follow-up appointment should be scheduled for 1 to 2 weeks in the future.

Beyond delivering MNT for GDM, registered dietitians may also incorporate the following into the first session:

- An explanation of GDM, including the diagnostic criteria and the risks to the woman and infant
- An explanation of the role of good nutrition in pregnancy
- An explanation of food portions and food groups, using food models and labels
- A demonstration of self-monitoring of blood glucose levels or ketone testing
- Assessment of the woman's comprehension of her MNT, her desire to follow the meal plan, and barriers to achieving clinical and educational outcomes
- Instruction about use of insulin or oral agent therapy in management of GDM

Finally, the registered dietitian should document the session in the medical record and complete billing forms and other forms as required.

Follow-Up Sessions

At the follow-up session(s), the registered dietitian should assess blood glucose values, weight change, and actual food intake. In addition, the woman's comprehension of and

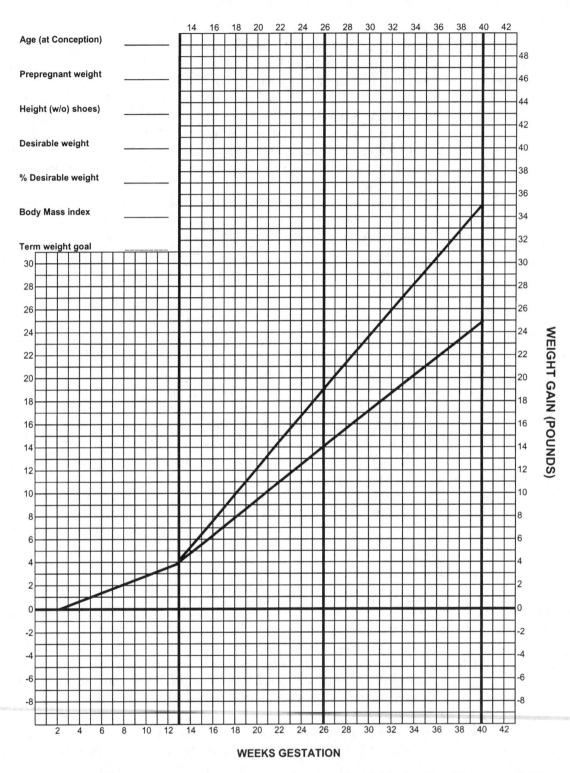

Age (at Conception) _____

Prepregnant weight _____

Height (w/o) shoes) _____

Desirable weight _____

% Desirable weight _____

Body Mass index _____

Term weight goal _____

WEIGHT GAIN (POUNDS)

WEEKS GESTATION

Note: Young adolescents, African American women, and smokers should strive for gains at the upper end of the recommended ranges. Short women (<62 inches) should strive for gains at the lower end of the range.

California Department of Health Services, MCH/WIC. Nutrition during Pregnancy and Postpartum Period, 6/90

FIGURE 6.2.   Prenatal weight gain grid for normal weight women. Reprinted from California Department of Health Services, MCH/WIC. Prenatal weight gain grids. Available at: http://www.sonoma-county.org/health/ph/chs_mch_coord/pdf/form_weight.pdf. Accessed December 28, 2004.

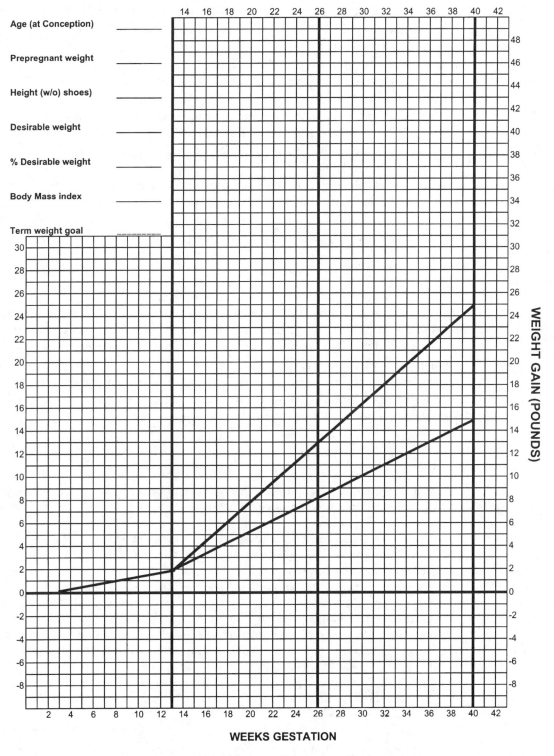

FIGURE 6.3. Prenatal weight gain grid for overweight women. Reprinted from California Department of Health Services, MCH/WIC. Prenatal weight gain grids. Available at: http://www.sonoma-county.org/health/ph/chs_mch_coord/pdf/form_weight.pdf. Accessed December 28, 2004.

ability to follow the food plan and other self-monitoring activities should be evaluated (2). The registered dietitian should adjust the diet plan, as needed, to ensure appropriate weight gain, good nutrition, and blood glucose values within the target range. If all these clinical outcomes cannot be achieved with MNT alone, then referral for additional therapy is appropriate. To see specific examples of GDM cases and the steps and forms used by dietetics professionals, see Appendix B.

The registered dietitian should discuss infant feeding plans. Pregnant women can benefit from information about breastfeeding even if they do not plan to breastfeed their babies. Appropriate referrals (eg, Special Supplemental Nutrition Program for Women, Infants, and Children [WIC], food resources, breastfeeding resources) should be offered.

Postpartum care, including support for breastfeeding and maternal weight reduction, is also recommended for women with GDM. Because women with GDM have a high risk for developing type 2 diabetes, information regarding prevention of diabetes should be presented (see Chapter 10).

SUMMARY

The cornerstone of treatment for women with GDM is MNT. MNT begins with an assessment of a woman's nutritional, maternal, and physical history. The registered dietitian then develops a food plan that promotes normoglycemia, appropriate maternal weight gain, and the nutrient needs of pregnancy, and the woman is taught how to follow this plan. Follow-up appointments are critical parts of MNT, because they provide the opportunity to assess whether implementation of the food plan meets clinical outcomes or whether pharmacologic therapy is needed. Postpartum follow-up is also recommended.

REFERENCES

1. Identifying patients at risk: ADA's definitions for nutrition screening and nutrition assessment. Council on Practice (COP) Quality Management Committee. *J Am Diet Assoc.* 1994;94:838–839.

2. American Dietetic Association. *Medical Nutrition Therapy Evidence-Based Guides for Practice: Nutrition Practice Guidelines for Gestational Diabetes Mellitus* [CD-ROM]. Chicago, Ill: American Dietetic Association; 2001.

3. American Dietetic Association. *Medical Nutrition Therapy Evidence-Based Guides for Practice: Nutrition Practice Guidelines Type 1 and Type 2 Diabetes Mellitus* [CD-ROM]. Chicago, Ill: American Dietetic Association; 2001.

4. deVeciana M, Major CA, Morgan MA, Asrat T, Toohey JS, Lien JM, Evans AT. Postprandial versus preprandial blood glucose monitoring in women with gestational diabetes requiring insulin therapy. *N Engl J Med.* 1995;333:1237–1241.

5. Metzger B, Coustan DC. Summary and recommendations of the Fourth International Workshop-Conference on Gestational Diabetes Mellitus. The Organizing Committee. *Diabetes Care.* 1998;21(suppl 2):B161–B167.

6. Jovanovic L, ed. *Medical Management of Pregnancy Complicated by Diabetes.* 3rd ed. Alexandria, Va. American Diabetes Association; 2000.

7. Gunderson EP. Intensive nutrition therapy for gestational diabetes. Rationale and current issues. *Diabetes Care.* 1997;20:221–226.

8. Institute of Medicine. *Dietary Reference Intakes for Energy, Carbohydrate, Fiber, Fat, Fatty Acids, Cholesterol, Protein, and Amino Acids (Macronutrients).* Washington, DC: National Academy Press; 2002.

9. Institute of Medicine. *Nutrition During Pregnancy: Part I: Weight Gain, Part II: Nutrient Supplements.* Washington, DC: National Academy Press; 1990.

10. Buchanan TA. Metabolic changes during normal and diabetic pregnancies. In: Reece EA, Coustan DR, eds. *Diabetes Mellitus in Pregnancy.* 2nd ed. New York, NY: Churchill Livingstone; 1995:59–77.

11. Kitzmiller JL, Gavin LA, Gin GD, Jovanovic-Peterson L, Main EK, Zigrang WD. Preconception care of diabetes. Glycemic control prevents congenital anomalies. *JAMA.* 1991;265:731–736.

12. Franz MJ, Bantle JP, Beebe CA, Brunzell JD, Chiasson JL, Garg A, Holzmeister LA, Hoogwerf B, Mayer-Davis E, Mooradian AD, Purnell JS, Wheeler M. Evidence-based nutrition principles and recommendations for the treatment and prevention of diabetes and related complications. *Diabetes Care.* 2002;25:148–198.

13. Sheard NF, Clark NG, Brand-Miller JC, Franz MJ, Pi-Sunyer FX, Mayer-Davis E, Kulkarni K, Geil P. Dietary carbohydrate (amount and type) in the prevention and management of diabetes: a statement by the American Diabetes Association. *Diabetes Care.* 2004;27:2266–2271.

14. Wahqluist ML, Wilmshurst EG, Richardson EN. The effect of chain length on glucose absorption and the related metabolic response. *Am J Clin Nutr.* 1978;31:1998–2001.

15. Foster-Powell K, Miller JB. International tables of glycemic index. *Am J Clin Nutr.* 1995;62(suppl):871S–890S.

16. Foster-Powell K, Holt SH, Brand-Miller JC. International table of glycemic index and glycemic load values: 2002. *Am J Clin Nutr.* 2002;76:5–56.

17. Perlstein RWJ, Hines C, Milsavljevic M. Dietitians Association of Australia review paper. Glycaemic index in diabetes management. *Nutr Diet.* 1997;54:57–63.

18. Canadian Diabetes Association. Guidelines for the nutritional management of diabetes mellitus in the new millennium. *Can J Diabetes.* 1999;23:56–69.

19. Recommendations for the nutritional management of patients with diabetes mellitus. *Eur J Clin Nutr.* 2000;54:353–355.

20. National Heart, Lung, and Blood Institute. Body mass index table. Available at: http://www.nhlbi.nih.gov/guidelines/obesity/bmi_tbl.htm. Accessed March 16, 2005.

21. National Heart, Lung, and Blood Institute. The Practical Guide: Identification, Evaluation, and Treatment of Overweight and Obesity in Adults. Available at: http://www.nhlbi.nih.gov/guidelines/obesity/prctgd_b.pdf. Accessed March 16, 2005.

22. Institute of Medicine. *Recommended Dietary Allowances.* 10th ed. Washington, DC: National Academy Press; 1989.

23. California Diabetes and Pregnancy Program. Guidelines for Care. Sacramento, Calif: Maternal and Child Health Branch, Department of Health Services; 2002.

24. Barr SI, Murphy SP, Poos MI. Interpreting and using the dietary references intakes in dietary assessment of individuals and groups. *J Am Diet Assoc.* 2002;102:780–788.

25. Institute of Medicine. *Dietary Reference Intakes for Vitamin A, Vitamin K, Arsenic, Boron, Chromium, Copper, Iodine, Iron, Manganese, Molybdenum, Nickel, Silicon, Vanadium, and Zinc.* Washington, DC: National Academy Press; 2001.

26. Institute of Medicine. *Dietary Reference Intakes for Calcium, Phosphorus, Magnesium, Vitamin D, and Fluoride.* Washington, DC: National Academy Press; 1997.

27. Institute of Medicine. *Dietary Reference Intakes for Vitamin C, Vitamin E, Selenium, and Carotenoids.* Washington, DC: National Academy Press; 2000.

28. Institute of Medicine. *Dietary Reference Intakes for Thiamin, Riboflavin, Niacin, Vitamin B6, Folate, Vitamin B12, Pantothenic Acid, Biotin, and Choline.* Washington, DC: National Academy Press; 2000.

29. Lichtenstein AH. Dietary fat and cardiovascular disease risk: quantity or quality? *J Womens Health (Larchmt).* 2003;12:109–114.

30. Kaplan JS, Iqbal S, England BG, Zawacki CM, Herman WH. Is pregnancy in diabetic women associated with folate deficiency? *Diabetes Care.* 1999;22:1017–1021.

31. Vollset SE, Refsum H, Irgens LM, Emblem BM, Tverdal A, Gjessing HK, Monsen AL, Ueland PM. Plasma total homocysteine, pregnancy complications, and adverse pregnancy outcomes: the Hordaland Homocysteine study. *Am J Clin Nutr.* 2000;71:962–968.

32. Recker RR, Davies KM, Hinders SM, Heaney RP, Stegman MR, Kimmel DB. Bone gain in young adult women. *JAMA.* 1992;268:2403–2408.

33. Heaney RP, Abrams S, Dawson-Hughes B, Looker A, Marcus R, Matkovic V, Weaver C. Peak bone mass. *Osteoporos Int.* 2000;11:985–1009.

34. Pollitzer WS, Anderson JJ. Ethnic and genetic differences in bone mass: a review with a hereditary vs environmental perspective. *Am J Clin Nutr.* 1989;50:1244–1259.

35. Smith DM, Nance WE, Kang KW, Christian JC, Johnston CC Jr. Genetic factors in determining bone mass. *J Clin Invest.* 1973;52:2800–2808.

36. Richie LD, King JC. Dietary calcium and pregnancy induced hypertension: is there a relation? *Am J Clin Nutr.* 2000;71(suppl):1371S–1374S.

37. King JC. The risk of maternal nutritional depletion and poor outcomes increases in early or closely spaced pregnancies. *J Nutr.* 2003;133(Suppl 2):1732S–1736S.

38. Kaiser LL, Allen L, American Dietetic Association. Position of the American Dietetic Association: nutrition and lifestyle for a healthy pregnancy outcome. *J Am Diet Assoc.* 2002;102:1479–1490.

39. American Dietetic Association and Dietitians of Canada. Position of the American Dietetic Association and Dietitians of Canada: vegetarian diets. *J Am Diet Assoc.* 2003;103:748–765.

40. Sanders TA. The nutritional adequacy of plant-based diets. *Proc Nutr Soc.* 1999;58:265–269.

41. Drake R, Reddy S, Davies J. Nutrient intake during pregnancy and pregnancy outcome of lacto-ovo-vegetarians, fish-eaters and non-vegetarians. *Veg Nutr.* 1998;2:45–52.

42. Mangels R. Vegetarian nutrition during pregnancy and lactation. *Perinat Nutr Rep.* 1997;4:1–4.

43. Mangels R. Vegetarian diets during pregnancy. *Issues in Vegetarian Dietetics.* 1999;9:1,4–8.

44. Klebanoff MA, Levine RJ, DerSimonian R, Clemens JD, Wilkins DG. Maternal serum paraxanthine, a caffeine metabolite, and the risk of spontaneous abortion. *N Engl J Med.* 1999;341:1639–1644.

45. Cnattingius S, Signorelo LB, Anneren G Clausson B, Ekbom A, Ljunger E, Blot W, McLaughlin JK, Petersson G, Rane A, Granath F. Caffeine intake and the risk of first-trimester spontaneous abortion. *N Engl J Med.* 2000;343:1839–1845.

46. Hatch EE, Bracken MB. Association of delayed conception with caffeine consumption. *Am J Epidemiol.* 1993;138:1082–1092.

47. Pitkin RM, Reynolds WA, Filer LJ Jr, Kling TG. Placental transmission and fetal distribution of saccharin. *Am J Obstet Gynecol.* 1971;111:280–286.

48. National Cancer Institute. Cancer Facts: Artificial Sweeteners. Available at: http://cis.nci.nih.gov/fact/pdfdraft/3_risk/fs3_19.pdf. Accessed March 16, 2005.

49. American Dietetic Association. Position of the American Dietetic Association: use of nutritive and nonnutritive sweeteners. *J Am Diet Assoc.* 2004;104:255–275.

50. California Department of Health Services, MCH/WIC. Prenatal Weight Gain Grids. Available at: http://www.sonoma-county.org/health/ph/chs_mch_coord/pdf/form_weight.pdf. Accessed March 16, 2005.

51. American Dietetic Association and American Diabetes Association. *Basic Carbohydrate Counting.* Chicago, Ill: American Dietetic Association; 2003.

52. International Diabetes Center. *My Food Plan for Gestational Diabetes.* Minneapolis, Minn: International Diabetes Center; 2003.

53. International Diabetes Center. *Gestational Diabetes: Caring for Yourself and Your Baby.* Minneapolis, Minn: International Diabetes Center; 2001.

7

Medications and Supplements

Alyce M. Thomas, RD

OBJECTIVES   After completing this chapter, you will be able to do the following:

1. Summarize the types, action, peak times, and duration of insulin used in pregnancy.
2. Explain treatment modalities used for hypoglycemia.
3. Describe possible uses of oral agents to treat diabetes in pregnancy.
4. Discuss the reasons for recommending use of multivitamin-mineral supplements in pregnancy.
5. Evaluate the benefits and adverse effects of herbal and botanical supplements on pregnancy outcome.

INSULIN

Medical nutrition therapy (MNT) is the appropriate treatment for gestational diabetes mellitus (GDM) if it allows the woman with GDM to maintain a fasting blood glucose level ≤95 mg/dL (5.3 mmol/L) and a 2-hour postprandial glucose level ≤120 mg/dL (6.7 mmol/L). The American Diabetes Association recommends the initiation of insulin therapy when MNT alone cannot maintain a fasting blood glucose level of 105 mg/dL (5.8 mmol/L), a 1-hour postprandial glucose level ≤155 mg/dL (8.6 mmol/L), or a 2-hour postprandial glucose level ≤130 mg/dL (7.2 mmol/L) (1).

However, not all clinicians follow this recommendation (2). To prevent fetal macrosomia, some clinicians aggressively treat hyperglycemia through the prophylactic use of insulin in all women with GDM (3). Others use ultrasound measurement of the fetal abdominal circumference, to determine whether insulin therapy is appropriate (4,5). Kjos et al (4) compared fetal outcomes of 98 women with fasting plasma glucose levels of 105 to

120 mg/dL (5.8 to 6.7 mmol/L) randomized into two groups: a control group on insulin therapy and an experimental group in which insulin was initiated only if the fetal abdominal circumference was greater than the 70th percentile and/or the fasting plasma glucose value was greater than 120 mg/dL (6.7 mmol/L). The experimental group received monthly ultrasounds. All subjects received MNT. There were no significant differences between the birth weights, frequencies of birth weights greater than the 90th percentile, or incidence of neonatal morbidity between the two groups. Women in the experimental group who did not receive insulin had infants with lower birth weights than did women on insulin (4).

In most cases, health care practitioners should wait 1 to 2 weeks after the initiation of MNT, to determine whether insulin must be administered to lower blood glucose levels to fall within target ranges (6–9).

Administration

When on insulin therapy, women with GDM must be willing to self-administer insulin several times daily. Dietetics professionals can encourage insulin therapy by educating women on topics such as peak times, the relationship between food and insulin action, and correct insulin storage and injection practices. Insulin does not require refrigeration, and it should not be stored at extreme temperatures. The woman must be instructed on how to measure and/or mix insulin doses and on proper techniques for needle and syringe disposal. The practice of reusing needles should be discouraged. In addition to needles and syringes, other devices used to administer insulin include jet injectors and insulin pens (10).

Women with GDM should demonstrate their proficiency at drawing up and injecting insulin. The woman should check each insulin vial for the expiration date and to ensure that the insulin is the correct type (11). Once a vial is opened, the potency of the insulin may be reduced after a month (12). If necessary, the vial is gently rolled to re-suspend the insulin. If a combination of short- and intermediate-acting insulin is used, the short-acting insulin should always be drawn up first. Air bubbles, which can contribute to an inaccurate measurement of the injection dose, must be eliminated.

Injections should be made in subcutaneous tissue and never in muscle. The woman should notify her physician or diabetes educator if there is any bruising, swelling, or pain at the injection site. If bruising occurs, the affected area should not be used for more injections until it has healed. The abdomen has the quickest rate of absorption. If the woman is unwilling to inject herself in the abdomen, other recommended sites are the thighs, arms, and buttocks (12). Injection sites should be rotated, to avoid the development of lipohypertrophy or lipoatrophy. The American Diabetes Association recommends rotating sites within one area of the body, because absorption rates vary from one part of the body to another (1).

Types of Insulin

Insulin is available in two forms: pork insulin and recombinant human insulin. Recombinant human insulin is recommended during pregnancy, because it is less allergenic than animal-based insulin (10–12). Use of human insulin in pregnancy is also advantageous because it has a more rapid onset and shorter duration than pork insulin (10,13).

As shown in Table 7.1 (9,14–16), several types of insulin are available: rapid-acting, short-acting, intermediate-acting, and long-acting. For a list of manufacturers of human insulin, see Table 7.2.

TABLE 7.1   Action of Human Insulin

Insulin Type	Onset, h	Peak Action, h	Duration, h
Rapid-acting (lispro, aspart)	0.08–0.25 (5–15 min)	1–2	4–6
Short-acting (regular)	0.5–1	2–4	3–10
Intermediate (NPH, lente)	1–2	4–8	10–20
Long-acting			
Ultralente	2–4	Unpredictable	16–20
Glargine (Lantus)	1–2	Flat	24

Source: Data are from references 9 and 14–16.

Rapid Acting

Rapid-acting insulin analogs (aspart or lispro) are used to reduce postprandial glucose concentrations. Rapid-acting insulin analogs are created by modifying two amino acids within the insulin molecule. This modification increases the insulin absorption rate and the peak serum insulin concentration. The onset (5 to 15 minutes), peak action (1 to 2 hours), and duration (4 to 6 hours) of rapid-acting insulin are shorter than in short-acting insulin (12,14,16,17).

Lispro and aspart can be injected at the beginning of a meal or immediately after, whereas short-acting insulin must be administered 30 minutes before a meal. Rapid-acting insulin has not been found to cross the placenta, and its use in pregnancy has increased during the last 5 years (17–21). In a study involving 42 women with GDM randomized into two groups (lispro vs short-acting insulin), lispro was associated with fewer hypoglycemic episodes (19). The Food and Drug Administration has classified lispro as Category B. This category indicates that (*a*) animal-reproduction studies have not demonstrated a fetal risk but there are no controlled studies in pregnant women, or (*b*) animal-reproduction studies have shown an adverse effect (other than a decrease in fertility) that was not confirmed in controlled studies in women in the first trimester (and no evidence of a risk in later trimesters) (22).

Short-Acting

Short-acting insulin (also known as regular insulin) is usually injected 30 minutes before a meal. The onset is within 30 to 60 minutes; action peaks in 2 to 4 hours; and duration is 6 to 10 hours (14). A woman should not eat immediately after injecting short-acting insulin, because eating reduces the insulin action that prevents glycemic levels from rising too rapidly. Optimal times for insulin injections and meals must be individualized and depend on several factors, such as injection site or physical activity (16). The peak action of the insulin may be delayed as it travels from subcutaneous tissue to the bloodstream (10). Women taking short-acting insulin should eat snacks, because hypoglycemia may occur between meals (9,23).

Intermediate-Acting

Neutral protamine Hagedorn (NPH) insulin is an intermediate-acting insulin, which is often used in pregnancy (20). Its onset is 2 to 4 hours after injecting, action peaks in 4 to 12 hours, and its duration is 10 to 18 hours (14). NPH is usually given twice daily: before breakfast to cover the lunch meal and at bedtime to avoid nocturnal hypoglycemia. Inter-

TABLE 7.2 Manufacturers of Human Insulin (U-100)

Product	Manufacturer*
Rapid-acting (onset <15 min)	
Humalog (insulin lispro)	Lilly
Humalog Cartridge (3 mL & 1.5 mL)	Lilly
Humalog Prefilled Pen (3 mL)	Lilly
NovoLog PenFill (insulin aspart) (3 mL)	Lilly
NovoLog (insulin aspart)	Lilly
Short-acting (onset 30 min–2 h)	
Humulin R (regular)	Lilly
Novolin R (regular)	Novo Nordisk
Novolin R PenFill (3mL)	Novo Nordisk
Intermediate-acting (onset 2–4 h)	
Humulin L (lente)	Lilly
Humulin N (NPH)	Lilly
Humulin N Prefilled Pen (3 mL)	Lilly
Novolin L (lente) Novo Nordisk	Lilly
Novolin N (NPH) Novo Nordisk	Novo Nordisk
Novolin N PenFill (3 mL)	Novo Nordisk
Long-acting	
Humulin U (Ultralente) (onset 4–6 hours)	Lilly
Glargine (insulin glargine) (onset 1.1 hours)	Aventis Pharmaceuticals
Combinations	
Humulin 50/50 (50% NPH, 50% regular)	Lilly
Humulin 60/30 (70% NPH, 30% regular)	Lilly
Humulin 70/30 Prefilled Pen (3 mL) (70% NPH, 30% regular)	Lilly
Humalog Mix 75/25 (75% insulin lispro protamine suspension & 25% insulin lispro rDNA origin)	Lilly
Humalog 75/25 Prefilled Pen (3 mL)	Lilly
Novolin 70/30 (70% NPH, 30% NPH)	Novo Nordisk
Novolin 70/30 PenFill (70% NPH, 30% regular, 3 mL)	Novo Nordisk
NovoLog Mix 70/30 (70% insulin aspart [rDNA origin] protamine suspension & 30% insulin aspart [rDNA origin] injection	Novo Nordisk

*Avenits, Bridgewater, NJ 08807–2854; Eli Lilly and Company, Indianapolis, IN 46285; Novo Nordisk, Princeton, NJ 08540.

Source: Adapted with permission from Diabetes Care and Education Dietetic Practice Group. *American Dietetic Association Guide to Diabetes Medical Nutrition Therapy and Education.* Chicago, Ill: American Dietetic Association; 2005.

mediate-acting insulin before dinner should not be injected, because the peak action time will occur during the middle of the night and cause overnight glucose excursions.

Long-Acting

Ultralente is a long-acting insulin and is usually effective for 10 to 16 hours. It is not often used in pregnancy and is prescribed primarily in the presence of significant insulin resistance. The response of a long-acting insulin may not meet rapid insulin needs during pregnancy (15). However, ultralente may be useful if high doses of intermediate-acting insulin are required for euglycemia. A study comparing short- and long-acting insulin found improved blood glucose control and a decrease in the incidence of neonatal complications with short-acting insulin (24).

Glargine (Lantus; Aventis Pharmaceuticals, Kansas City, MO 64137) is another long-acting basal insulin analog. It is produced by adding two arginine molecules to recombinant DNA, which delays the action of the insulin, with no peak action time. Glargine is usually administered at bedtime, but it can be given at any time during the day. There are few studies on the use and effects of glargine in pregnancy, and the FDA has classified this drug in Category C (19,20). This category indicates that (*a*) studies in animals have revealed adverse effects on the fetus (teratogenic or embryocidal or other) and there are no controlled studies in women, or (*b*) studies in animals are not available. Drugs in this category should be given only if the potential benefit justifies the potential risk to the fetus (22).

Calculating Insulin Requirements

Insulin requirements increase throughout pregnancy. The amount of insulin to be administered for GDM in the first trimester is 0.6 to 0.8 U/kg body weight; in the second trimester, the insulin requirement is 1.0 U/kg body weight; and in the third trimester, the requirement is 1.2 U/kg body weight (25).

Insulin therapy in GDM varies. The most common insulin plan combines short- and intermediate-acting insulin (10,17,26). See Figure 7.1 (27) for a representation of this plan. A midmorning snack may be necessary to avoid late-morning hypoglycemia. Intermediate-acting insulin is injected at bedtime, and not at dinner, to avoid hypoglycemia in the middle of the night. Adjustments in the insulin plan depend on blood glucose levels (10).

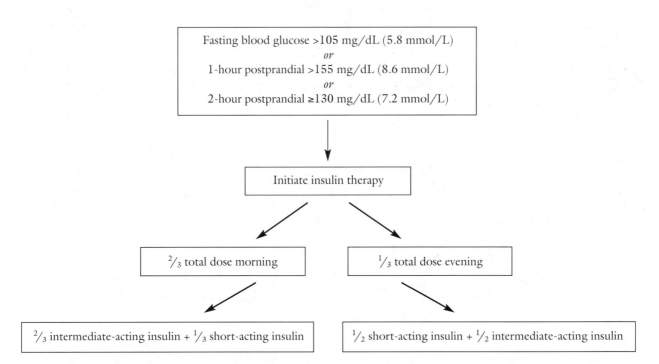

FIGURE 7.1. Using intermediate- and short-acting insulins. Reprinted with permission from Jones MW, Stone LC. Management of the woman with gestational diabetes mellitus. *J Perinat Neonat Nurs.* 1998;11:13–24.

Selected Multiple-Insulin-Injection Plans

Rapid-Acting and NPH Insulin

As shown in Figure 7.2 (28), in insulin therapy combining rapid-acting and NPH insulin, rapid-acting insulin is injected before breakfast and dinner, whereas NPH is given at bedtime, to provide glucose control overnight and to prevent early-morning hyperglycemia, and at breakfast, to provide a basal rate throughout the day and to cover lunch. Meals must be eaten on time to avoid hypoglycemia.

Short-Acting and NPH Insulin

In a plan combining short-acting and NPH insulin (Figure 7.3), short-acting insulin is used to cover breakfast and dinner (28). The NPH dose is given before bedtime. This timing of the NPH dose controls blood glucose levels during the night better than NPH taken at dinner. A disadvantage of this plan is that the lunch meal must be eaten on time. Although they are not shown in Figure 7.3, between-meal snacks can be added to this plan.

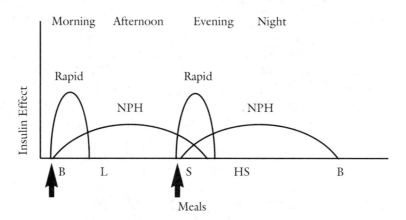

FIGURE 7.2. Using rapid-acting and NPH insulins. Reprinted with permission from American Diabetes Association. *Practical Insulin: A Handbook for Prescribers.* Alexandria, Va: American Diabetes Association; 2002.

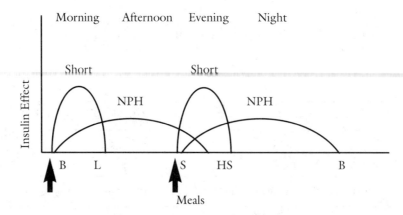

FIGURE 7.3. Using short-acting and NPH insulins. Reprinted with permission from American Diabetes Association. *Practical Insulin: A Handbook for Prescribers.* Alexandria, Va: American Diabetes Association; 2002.

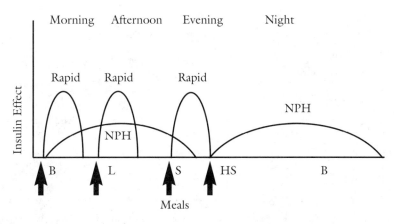

FIGURE 7.4. Using rapid-acting and intermediate-acting insulins. Reprinted with permission from American Diabetes Association. *Practical Insulin: A Handbook for Prescribers.* Alexandria, Va: American Diabetes Association; 2002.

Rapid-Acting and Intermediate-Acting Insulin

As shown in Figure 7.4 (28), the combination of rapid- and intermediate-acting insulin requires injections of short-acting insulin before three meals and two injections of intermediate-acting insulin: one at breakfast and the other at bedtime. Intermediate-acting insulin is used at night to reduce the risk of nocturnal hypoglycemia. A morning dose of NPH before breakfast provides daytime basal insulin. The rapid-acting insulin covers postprandial glucose excursions.

Ultralente and Rapid-acting or Short-acting Insulin

In this insulin plan, ultralente is used to provide basal insulin during the day and overnight and is usually administered at bedtime. Rapid- or short-acting insulin is given before each meal, to cover postmeal blood glucose excursions. This plan allows the person to adjust the insulin dose at mealtime based on postmeal blood glucose levels and meal composition.

Insulin-to-Carbohydrate Ratios

Carbohydrate counting may be used in GDM if insulin therapy is initiated. The ratio of carbohydrate to insulin is usually 1:15 when rapid-acting or short-acting insulin is used. However, the ratio may be lower at breakfast, because levels of hormonal activity are higher in the early morning hours (8). The insulin-to-carbohydrate ratio is also affected by body weight and by insulin resistance. For example, insulin-to-carbohydrate ratios may be lower in obese women (eg, 1:10) (15). For guidelines on calculating insulin-to-carbohydrate ratios using the 500/450 Rule or the Insulin Sensitivity Factor, see Box 7.1 (29).

Hypoglycemia

Hypoglycemia rarely occurs when GDM is controlled by MNT only. Hypoglycemia may occur in women who use insulin therapy or oral agents if they skip or delay a meal, if they exercise without consuming sufficient calories, or if they consume less food than what was prescribed on the meal plan. Hypoglycemia may also be caused by increased insulin absorption rates. In pregnancy, hypoglycemia may occur when a woman experiences nausea and vomiting (15).

BOX 7.1

Calculating Insulin-to-Carbohydrate Ratios

500/450 RULE

Take the daily insulin dose (TDD) and divide by 500. For example: if TDD is 50 units, then the insulin-to-carbohydrate ratio is 1:10 (1 unit of insulin is required for 10 g carbohydrate).

If the woman demonstrates insulin resistance, then divide the TDD by 450.

INSULIN SENSITIVITY FACTOR (ISF)

To calculate the ISF, divide 1,800 by TDD to determine the amount (in mg/dL) that 1 unit of insulin will lower blood glucose, then multiply that result by 0.33. For example, if TDD equals 50 units, dividing 1,800 by 50 equals 36 (1 unit insulin will lower blood glucose 36 mg/dL). Multiplying 36 by 0.33 provides an ISF of 11.8 (rounded up to 12). One unit insulin is required for each 12 g carbohydrate consumed, or an insulin-to-carbohydrate ratio of 1:12.

For insulin resistance, use 1,500 instead of 1,800.

Source: Data are from reference 29.

Diabetes educators and dietetics professionals should instruct women to follow the guidelines in Box 7.2 (9,10), to avoid hypoglycemia. Women with GDM should be taught the signs and symptoms of hypoglycemia, which include hunger, dizziness, feeling faint, headache, drowsiness, trembling, or irritability. If the woman experiences any of these symptoms, her blood glucose level must be checked before she is treated for hypoglycemia.

OTHER TREATMENT MODALITIES FOR HYPOGLYCEMIA

Oral Agents

Until recently, the use of oral agents for glycemic control was contraindicated in pregnancy, because of possible teratogenic effects and neonatal hypoglycemia (17,20,30). The first-generation sulfonylureas were found to cross the placental barrier and stimulate fetal insulin secretion, which caused fetal hyperinsulinemia (20,30). However, newer medications, such as second-generation sulfonylureas, which stimulate the pancreas to secrete insulin, do not significantly cross the placenta. Although the use of oral agents in pregnancy is not widespread, some clinicians advocate their use as an alternative to insulin (31–33). As a general rule, oral agents are less costly and are considered less invasive than insulin (31). In a study comparing the cost of the two types of medication, subjects using oral agents spent approximately $166 less than subjects using insulin (34).

Glyburide

Glyburide (Micronase, Diabeta; Pharmacia & Upjohn Company, Kalamazoo, MI 49001) is a second-generation sulfonylurea that may be an appropriate medication for women with GDM. It is minimally transported across the placental barrier and is not associated with neonatal hypoglycemia (25). Glyburide acts to improve glycemic control by stimulating the pancreas to increase insulin secretion (31). In a landmark randomized controlled study, Langer et al compared the use of glyburide with the use of insulin in GDM (35). There were no differences in the incidence of preeclampsia, cesarean deliveries, macrosomia, or anomalies between the two groups. No detectable levels of glyburide were found in umbilical cord samples. Although eight women from the glyburide group were eventually

BOX 7.2

Treatment Recommendations for Hypoglycemia

If the blood glucose is < 60 mg/dL, the treatment consists of consuming at least 15 g of carbohydrate and rechecking the blood glucose levels in 15 minutes. This regimen should be repeated if the levels remain below 60 mg/dL. If the hypoglycemia occurs within 30 minutes of a meal or snack, the woman should eat sooner. All women on insulin therapy or oral agents should be instructed to carry at least 15 g of carbohydrates with them in case of a hypoglycemic reaction.

The following contain 15 g carbohydrate:

- ½ cup orange juice
- ½ cup regular applesauce
- 4 ounces regular soda
- ½ cup regular flavored gelatin
- 6 saltines
- 1 cup soup
- ¼ cup sherbet
- ½ cup ice cream or frozen yogurt
- 3–4 glucose tablets
- 1 tablespoon sugar

The patient should be instructed on the use of readily available forms of glucose, such as tablets or gels.

Source: Data are from references 9 and 10.

switched to insulin to maintain blood glucose control, the researchers concluded that glyburide can be safely used in GDM. Other researchers have found similar results (33,36–38). The safety of glyburide in the first trimester of pregnancy is unknown.

Meal and snack adjustments are possible with glyburide treatment in GDM. Action of glyburide peaks 4 to 8 hours after it is taken, and it should be taken at least 30 to 60 minutes before meals. It may be necessary to add more frequent snacks and a larger amount of carbohydrate to the meal plan, because of the long half-life of glyburide (39).

Metformin

Metformin is a biguanide that works by decreasing hepatic glucose production, which improves peripheral glucose uptake and reduces insulin resistance. This oral agent crosses the placenta, but it has not been shown to cause neonatal hypoglycemia. A review article by Glueck et al noted no adverse effects with metformin therapy in GDM (40).

***

Additional research is recommended by the American College of Obstetricians and Gynecologists and others, before the use of oral agents in GDM is supported (30,41,42). For a summary of oral agents used in pregnancy, see Table 7.3 (43).

Continuous Subcutaneous Insulin Infusion

Continuous subcutaneous insulin infusion (CSII) is an effective alternative to multiple insulin injections in the treatment of diabetes (14). Rapid-acting insulin is continuously administered (basal) with boluses, to cover meals and snacks. A very-fine-gauge needle or cannula is inserted under the skin and is attached by plastic tubing to a pump. The cannula is reimplanted at a different site every 2 to 3 days. The amount of insulin used in the basal rate is 50% to 60% of the total; the rest is given as boluses. The largest bolus (30% to 35% of

TABLE 7.3 Oral Agents Used in Pregnancy

Class	Generic Name (Brand Name)	Indications	Adverse Effects	Comments
Sulfonylureas	Glyburide, micronized (Glynase PresTab)	Stimulates the pancreas to secrete insulin	Hypoglycemia	Taken before meals
Biguanides	Metformin (Glucophage); long-acting metformin (Glucophage XR)	Decreases absorption of glucose in small intestine	Nausea, diarrhea, loss of appetite	May cause lactic acidosis; not recommended if kidney dysfunction

Source: Adapted with permission from Diabetes Care and Education Dietetic Practice Group. *American Dietetic Association Guide to Diabetes Medical Nutrition Therapy and Education.* Chicago, Ill: American Dietetic Association; 2005.

the insulin administered in boluses) is given at breakfast; 25% of the bolus insulin is given before both lunch and dinner; and 15% to 25% is administered before snacks (44). A typical basal rate provides a lower amount of insulin from 10 pm to 4 am, when the woman is asleep, and administers a higher amount from 4 am to 10 pm, when insulin resistance is most prevalent. The rate is individualized to meet specific needs and may decrease slightly during the day if a woman's activity level increases.

Insulin pump therapy is considered in the management of diabetes when multiple injections fail to control blood glucose levels. It can help to improve glycemic control, to avoid nocturnal hyperglycemia, and to increase flexibility in diet and lifestyle. Blood glucose levels must be tested preprandially and postprandially (16,45,46).

Most studies of CSII use in pregnant women have focused on women with preexisting diabetes (46–49). Only one study (50) has examined CSII in women with GDM. In this case-control study of multiethnic women with GDM in Australia, the outcomes for subjects using insulin pump therapy were compared with those of subjects on conventional insulin therapy. Improved glycemic control was observed with the insulin pump within the first week after its introduction. Subjects using insulin pump therapy had greater insulin requirements and increased weight gain compared with subjects in the control group, and their infants were more likely to be admitted to the neonatal intensive unit. However, these infants were not significantly heavier, and the women on insulin pump therapy did not experience more hypoglycemic episodes than their counterparts. The researchers concluded that insulin pump therapy is safe and effective in controlling blood glucose levels in GDM.

Complications associated with CSII include possible ketotic episodes, infections or inflammations at the needle site, hypoglycemia, and pump malfunction (14,16,45). Using an insulin pump and supplies is more expensive than multiple insulin injection therapy. The woman will need extensive education and training in the use of the insulin pump. Also, CSII requires health care providers experienced in the management of pump therapy (45).

TOCOLYTIC AGENTS

Tocolytic agents are pharmacologic agents used to inhibit preterm labor (15). Beta-sympathomimetics are used to decrease uterine contractions. However, beta-sympathomimetics can cause maternal hyperglycemia (15,51,52). Insulin is initiated if glycemic levels cannot be controlled by diet alone (15). Nifedipine, a calcium channel blocker, also causes maternal hyperglycemia. The mechanism of magnesium sulfate as a tocolytic agent is not fully understood, although it is thought to act as a calcium antagonist and to prevent muscle contractility (52). Neither magnesium sulfate nor prostaglandin synthesis inhibitors, such as indomethacin, causes hyperglycemia.

VITAMIN-MINERAL SUPPLEMENTATION

Since 1990, the Institute of Medicine has recommended that all pregnant women receive nutrition counseling, to assess their need for nutrient supplementation (53). Some women, including pregnant women with inadequate dietary intakes, those with multiple gestations, cigarette smokers, and those who use alcohol or drugs, may need a daily supplement if their nutrition needs are above the Reference Daily Intakes (53). A low-dose iron supplement (30 mg/day) is recommended for all pregnant women, beginning at the first prenatal visit (53). The Institute of Medicine recommends that women at nutritional risk in the second and third trimesters of pregnancy take a daily multivitamin and mineral supplement containing the following nutrients (54):

- Iron: 30 mg
- Zinc: 15 mg
- Copper: 2 mg
- Calcium: 250 mg
- Vitamin B-6: 2 mg
- Folate: 600 µg
- Vitamin C: 50 mg
- Vitamin D: 5 µg

HERBAL USE IN PREGNANCY

The use of herbal supplements for the treatment of ailments has proliferated in recent years (55). Pregnant women use these products as alternatives to traditional medicine. In a study of the use of prescription, over-the-counter, and herbal medicines in pregnancy, 45.2% of the women interviewed used herbal medication (56). In another survey, 13% of the pregnant women used some type of dietary supplement (57).

The use of herbal supplements in pregnancy, however, has not been studied extensively. No controlled studies have been conducted to determine their safety and efficacy (58). The risks to the fetus of many supplements are unknown. Moreover, women may choose not to share information about supplement use with health care providers. Incomplete information about a woman's supplement use increases the risk of potentially dangerous drug-nutrient or drug-drug interactions.

Blue cohosh, evening primrose oil, red raspberry leaves, and black cohosh are used to promote labor (59). However, these supplements are contraindicated in pregnancy. Blue cohosh may cause tachycardia and hypotension in the woman as well as neonatal congestive heart failure (60). Evening primrose oil is a rich source of n-6 fatty acids (59,60). Adequate levels of n-3 fatty acids are associated with decreased risks of preterm delivery and low-birth-weight infants. Low levels of n-3 fatty acids, with corresponding high levels of n-6 fatty acids, are associated with preterm labor, intrauterine growth retardation, and depression (61–63). Red raspberry leaves are used to stimulate the onset of labor. The use of large doses in early pregnancy is discouraged for this reason (60). Black cohosh in large doses may cause nausea, vomiting, and headaches (60).

BOX 7.3

Dietary Supplements Contraindicated in Pregnancy

- Agnus castus
- Aloe
- Angelica
- Apricot kernal
- Asafoetida
- Aristolchia
- Avens
- Black cohosh
- Blue cohosh
- Blue flag
- Bogbean
- Boldo
- Boneset
- Borage
- Broom
- Buchu
- Buckthorn
- Burdock
- Calamus
- Calendula
- Cascara
- Chaparral
- Cola
- Coltsfoot
- Comfrey
- Cottonroot
- Cornsilk
- Crotalaris
- Damiana
- Devil's claw
- Dong quai
- Dogbane
- Ephedra
- Eupatorium
- Euphorbia

- Fenugreek
- Feverfew
- Foxglove
- Fucus
- Gentian
- German chamomile
- Germander
- Ginseng
- Golden seal
- Ground ivy
- Grounsel
- Guarana
- Hawthorne
- Heliotropium
- Hops
- Horehound
- Horsetail
- Horseradish
- Hydrocotyle
- Jamaica dogwood
- Juniper
- Liferoot
- Licorice
- Lobelia
- Mandrake
- Mate
- Male fern
- Meadowsweet
- Melliot
- Mistletoe
- Motherwort
- Myrrh
- Nettle
- Osha
- Passionflower

- Pennyroyal
- Petasites
- Plantain
- Pleurisy root
- Podophyllium
- Pokeroot
- Poplar
- Prickly ash
- Pulsatilla
- Queen's delight
- Ragwort
- Raspberry
- Red Clover
- Rhubarb
- Roman chamomile
- Rue
- Sassafras
- Scullcap
- Senna
- Shepherd's purse
- Skunk cabbage
- Stephania
- Squill
- St. John's wort
- Tansy
- Tonka bean
- Uva-ursi
- Vervain
- Wild carrot
- Willow
- Wormwood
- Yarrow
- Yellow dock
- Yohimbe

Source: Adapted with permission from Kaiser LL, Allen L; American Dietetic Association. Position of the American Dietetic Association: nutrition and lifestyle for a healthy pregnancy outcome. *J Am Diet Assoc.* 2002;102:1479–1490.

Other common herbal supplements that are contraindicated in pregnancy include St. John's wort (it may induce abortion and is not recommended for individuals with severe depression), ginseng (it may cause uterine stimulation), and goldenseal (it causes uterine stimulation and hypotension) (57,59,60). For a more extensive list of herbal and botanical supplements contraindicated in pregnancy, see Box 7.3 (64).

SUMMARY

The goal in the management of GDM is normoglycemia. The first course of treatment is MNT. If plasma glucose levels cannot be maintained by MNT, insulin is initiated. Education is the key to successful self-administration of insulin. Several types of insulin are available: rapid-acting, short-acting, intermediate-acting, and long-acting.

As pregnancy progresses, insulin requirements increase. The most common insulin plan for GDM is a combination of short-acting and intermediate-acting insulin. The 500/450 Rule and the Insulin Sensitivity Factor are two ways to calculate insulin-to-carbohydrate ratios. Oral agents (glyburide, metformin) are less expensive and easier to administer than insulin and are possible alternatives to insulin therapy in GDM.

The routine use of multivitamin-mineral supplements is recommended in the second and third trimesters of pregnancy for women at nutritional risk (those with multiple gestations, those who smoke heavily, and those who use alcohol or illegal drugs). Nutrition assessment and counseling are recommended for all pregnant women.

Many women use herbal and botanical supplements during pregnancy, often without the knowledge of their health care providers. Certain supplements are contraindicated during pregnancy and may have adverse maternal and fetal effects, such as uterine stimulation, premature labor, fetal congestive heart failure, and intrauterine growth retardation in the fetus.

REFERENCES

1. American Diabetes Association. Gestational diabetes mellitus. *Diabetes Care*. 2004;27(Suppl 1):S88–S90.
2. Langer O. Maternal glycemic criteria for insulin therapy in gestational diabetes mellitus. *Diabetes Care*. 1998;21(Suppl 2):B91–B98.
3. Kjos, SL, Buchanan TA. Gestational diabetes mellitus. *N Engl J Med*. 1999;341:1749–1756.
4. Kjos SL, Schaefer-Graf U, Sardesi S, Peters RK, Buley A, Xiang AH, Bryne JD, Sutherland C, Montoro MN, Buchanan TA. A randomized controlled trial using glycemic plus ultrasound parameters versus glycemic parameters to determine insulin therapy in gestational diabetes with fasting hyperglycemia. *Diabetes Care*. 2001;24:1904–1910.
5. Schaefer-Graf UM, Kjos SL, Fauzan OH, Buhling KJ, Siebert G, Buhrer C, Ladendorf B, Dudenhausen JW, Vetter K. A randomized trial evaluating a predominately fetal growth-based strategy to guide management of gestational diabetes in Caucasian women. *Diabetes Care*. 2004;27:297–302.
6. Major CA. Diabetes and pregnancy. In: Gleicher N, Buttino L, Elksyam U, Evans MI, Galbraith RM, eds. *Principles and Practices of Medical Therapy in Pregnancy*. Stamford, Conn: Appleton and Lange; 1998:461–471.
7. McFarland MB, Langer O, Conway DL, Berkus MD. Dietary therapy for gestational diabetes: how long is long enough? *Obstet Gynecol*. 1999;93:978–982.
8. American Diabetes Association. Position statement. Gestational diabetes mellitus. *Diabetes Care*. 1996;19(Suppl 1):S29.
9. *American Dietetic Association Medical Nutrition Therapy Evidence-Based Guides for Practice: Nutrition Practice Guidelines for Gestational Diabetes Mellitus* [CD-ROM]. Chicago, Ill: American Dietetic Association; 2001.
10. American Diabetes Association. Insulin administration. *Diabetes Care*. 2004;27(Suppl 1):S106-S109.
11. Simon ER. Gestational diabetes mellitus: diagnosis, treatment, and beyond. *Diabetes Educ*. 2001;27:69–74.
12. Jones MW, Stone LC. Management of the woman with gestational diabetes mellitus. *J Perinat Neonat Nurs*. 1998;11:13–24.

13. Landon MB, Gabbe SG. Insulin treatment of the pregnant patient with diabetes mellitus. In: Reece EA, Cousan DR, eds. *Diabetes in Women: Adolescence, Pregnancy, and Menopause*. 3rd ed. Philadelphia, Pa: Lippincott Williams & Wilkins; 2004:257–272.

14. Franz MJ, ed. *Diabetes Management Therapies: A Core Curriculum for Diabetes Educators*. 5th ed. Chicago, Ill: American Association of Diabetes Educators; 2003.

15. Jovanovic L, ed. *Medical Management of Pregnancy Complicated by Diabetes*. 3rd ed. Alexandria, Va: American Diabetes Association; 2000.

16. Klingensmith GJ, ed. *Intensive Diabetes Management*. Alexandria, Va: American Diabetes Association; 2003.

17. Simmons D. The utility and efficacy of the new insulins in the management of diabetes and pregnancy. *Curr Diab Rep*. 2002;2:331–336.

18. Jovanovic L. Optimization of insulin therapy in patients with gestational diabetes. *Endocr Pract*. 2000;6:98–101.

19. Jovanovic L, Ilic S, Pettitt DJ, Hugo K, Gutierrez M, Bowsher RR, Bastyr EJ 3rd. Metabolic and immunologic effects of insulin lispro in gestational diabetes. *Diabetes Care*. 1999;22:1422–1427.

20. Jovanovic L. Controversies in the diagnosis and treatment of gestational diabetes. *Cleve Clin J Med*. 2000;67:481–482, 485–486, 488.

21. Pettitt DJ, Ospina P, Kolaczynski JW, Jovanovic L. Comparison of an insulin analog, insulin aspart, and regular human with no insulin in gestational diabetes mellitus. *Diabetes Care*. 2003;26:183–186.

22. US Food and Drug Administration. FDA Pregnancy Chart. Available at: http://medicalcorps .org/med-org/Meds/PregnancyCategories.htm. Accessed February 5, 2005.

23. Luke B. Dietary management. In: Reece EA, Cousan DR. eds. *Diabetes in Women: Adolescence, Pregnancy, and Menopause*. 3rd ed. Philadelphia, Pa: Lippincott Williams and Wilkins; 2004:273–282.

24. Pöyhönen-Alho M, Teramo K, Kaaja R. Treatment of gestational diabetes with short- or long-acting insulin and neonatal outcome: a pilot study. *Acta Obstet Gynecol Scand*. 2002;81:258–259.

25. Gabbe SG, Graves CR. Management of diabetes mellitus complicating pregnancy. *Obstet Gynecol*. 2003;102:857–868.

26. Turok DK, Ratcliffe SD, Baxley EG. Management of gestational diabetes mellitus. *Am Fam Physician*. 2003;68:1767–1772.

27. Jones MW, Stone LC. Management of the woman with gestational diabetes mellitus. *J Perinat Neonat Nurs*. 1998;11:13–24.

28. American Diabetes Association. *Practical Insulin: A Handbook for Prescribers*. Alexandria, Va: American Diabetes Association, 2002.

29. Bradley BA. Insulin-to-carbohydrate ratios: how are they calculated? *Diabetes Interview*. 2003(Feb):42–44.

30. American College of Obstetricians and Gynecologists Committee on Practice Bulletins—Obstetrics. ACOG Practice Bulletin. Clinical management guidelines for obstetrician-gynecologists. Number 30, September 2001 (replaces Technical Bulletin Number 200, December 1994). Gestational diabetes. *Obstet Gynecol*. 2001;98:525–538.

31. Langer O. Oral hypoglycemic agents and the pregnant diabetic: "from bench to bedside." *Semin Perinatol*. 2002;26:215–224.

32. Langer O, Yogev Y, Xenakis EM, Rosenn B. Insulin and glyburide therapy: dosage, severity level of gestational diabetes, and pregnancy outcome. *Am J Obstet Gynecol*. 2005;192:134–139.

33. Kremer CJ, Duff P. Glyburide for the treatment of gestational diabetes. *Am J Obstet Gynecol*. 2004;190:1438–1439.

34. Goetzl L, Wilkins I. Glyburide compared to insulin for the treatment of gestational diabetes mellitus: a cost analysis. *J Perinatol*. 2001;22:403–406.

35. Langer O, Conway DL, Berkus MD, Xenakis EM, Gonzales O. A comparison of glyburide and insulin in women with gestational diabetes mellitus. *N Engl J Med*. 2000;343:1134–1138.

36. Towner D, Kjos SL, Leung B, Montoro MM, Xiang A, Mestman JH, Buchanan TA. Congenital malformations in pregnancies complicated by NIDDM. *Diabetes Care.* 1995;18:1446–1451.

37. Elliott BD, Langer O, Schenker S, Johnson RF. Insignificant transfer of glyburide occurs across the human placenta. *Am J Obstet Gynecol.* 1991;165:807–812.

38. Conway DL, Gonzales O, Skiver D. Use of glyburide for the treatment of gestational diabetes: the San Antonio experience. *J Mater Fetal Neonatal Med.* 2004;15:51–55.

39. Fagen C. Glyburide use in gestational diabetes. *On the Cutting Edge.* 2002;2392:11–12.

40. Glueck CJ, Goldenberg N, Streicher P, Wang P. Metformin and gestational diabetes. *Curr Diab Rep.* 2003;3:303–312.

41. Slocum JM, Sosa ME. Use of antidiabetics agents in pregnancy: current practice and controversy. *J Perinat Neonatal Nurs.* 2002;16:40–53.

42. Merlob P, Levitt O, Stahl B. Oral antihyperglycemic agents during pregnancy and lactation: a review. *Paediatr Drugs.* 2002;4:755–760.

43. Diabetes Care and Education Dietetic Practice Group. *American Dietetic Association Guide to Diabetes Medical Nutrition Therapy and Education.* Chicago, Ill: American Dietetic Association; 2005.

44. Landon MD, Catalano PM, Gabbe SG. Diabetes mellitus. In: Gabbe SG, Niebyl JR, Simpson JL, eds. *Obstetrics: Normal and Problem Pregnancies.* 4th ed. New York, NY: Churchill Livingstone; 2002:1081–1116.

45. American Diabetes Association. Continuous subcutaneous insulin infusion. *Diabetes Care.* 2004;27(Suppl 1):S110.

46. El-Sayed YY, Lydell DJ. New therapies for the pregnant patient with diabetes. *Diabetes Technol Ther.* 2001;3:635–640.

47. Coustan DR, Reece EA, Sherwin RS, Rudolf MC, Bates SE, Sockin SM, Holford T, Tamborlane WV. A randomized clinical trial of the insulin pump vs intensive conventional therapy in diabetic pregnancies. *JAMA.* 1986;255:631–636.

48. Gabbe SG. New concepts and applications in the use of the insulin pump during pregnancy. *J Matern-Fetal Med.* 2000;9:42–45.

49. Caruso A, Lanzone A, Bianchi V, Massidda M, Castelli MP, Fulghesu AM, Mancuso S. Continuous subcutaneous insulin infusion (CSII) in pregnant diabetic patients. *Prenat Diag.* 1987;7:41–50.

50. Simmons D, Thompson CF, Conroy C Scott DJ. Use of insulin pumps in pregnancies complicated by type 2 diabetes and gestational diabetes in a multiethnic community. *Diabetes Care.* 2001;24:2078–2082.

51. Hollingsworth DR. *Pregnancy, Diabetes and Birth: A Management Guide.* 2nd ed. Baltimore, Md: Williams and Wilkins; 1992.

52. Iams JD, Creasy RK. Preterm labor and delivery. In: Creasy RK, Resnik R, Iams JD, eds. *Maternal-Fetal Medicine: Principles and Practice.* 5th ed. Philadelphia, Pa: Saunders; 2004:623–661.

53. Centers for Disease Control and Prevention. Recommendations to prevent and control iron deficiency in the United States. *MMWR.* 1998;47:1–36

54. Institute of Medicine. *Nutrition During Pregnancy.* Washington, DC: National Academy Press; 1990.

55. Tesch BJ. Herbs commonly used by women: an evidence-based review. *Clin J Womens Health.* 2001;1:89–102.

56. Glover DD, Amonkar M, Rybeck BF, Tracy TS. Prescription over-the-counter, and herbal medicine use in a rural, obstetric population. *Am J Obstet Gynecol.* 2003;188:1039–1045.

57. Tsui B, Dennehy CE, Tsourounis C. A survey of dietary supplement use during pregnancy at an academic medical center. *Am J Obstet Gynecol.* 2001;185:433–437.

58. Zick SM, Raisler J, Warber A. Pregnancy. *Clin Fam Pract.* 2002;4:2005.

59. Warber SL, Bancroft JM, Pedroza JM. Herbal appendix. *Clin Fam Pract.* 2002;1168–1173.

60. Stevens DL. The use of complementary and alternative therapies in diabetes. *Clin Fam Pract.* 2002;4:911.

61. Timonen M, Horrobin D, Jokelainen J, Laitinen J, Herva A, Rasanen P. Fish consumption and depression: the Northern Finland 1966 birth cohort study. *J Affect Disord.* 2004;82:447–452.

62. Saldeen P, Saldeen T. Women and omega-3 fatty acids. *Obstet Gynecol Surv.* 2004;59:722–730.

63. Gallagher S. Omegas 3 oils and pregnancy. *Midwifery Today Int Midwife.* 2004;69:26–31.

64. Kaiser LL, Allen L; American Dietetic Association. Position of the American Dietetic Association: nutrition and lifestyle for a healthy pregnancy outcome. *J Am Diet Assoc.* 2002;102:1479–1490.

Additional Concerns in Pregnancy Complicated by Gestational Diabetes Mellitus

Alyce M. Thomas, RD, and Yolanda M. Gutierrez, MS, PhD, RD

OBJECTIVES   After completing this chapter, you will be able to do the following:

1. Describe treatments to alleviate the symptoms of nausea and vomiting in pregnancy.
2. Discuss the effect of certain gastrointestinal discomforts in pregnancy.
3. List the guidelines and contraindications of exercise in gestational diabetes mellitus (GDM).
4. Explain the possible effects of GDM in adolescents.
5. Summarize the effects of substance use on the pregnant woman and her fetus.

NAUSEA AND VOMITING

Morning Sickness

Nausea and vomiting, which are often referred to as morning sickness, are two of the most common complications in pregnancy. Approximately 70% to 85% of pregnant American women experience these symptoms (1). A natural but little understood discomfort (2), morning sickness occurs in the early stages of pregnancy, beginning around the 4th to 6th week of gestation (3). The symptoms are usually mild, and in 80% of the cases they resolve by the 20th week of gestation (4).

The cause of morning sickness is not well understood. An elevated level of human chorionic gonadotropin (HCG) hormone in the first trimester may be a factor (5,6). Increased levels of estrogen or a progesterone deficiency have also been suggested as possible causes (1,3).

Women experiencing morning sickness are more likely to have favorable outcomes from their pregnancies than those without the symptoms (7). Studies have found a decreased risk of spontaneous abortions, low birth weight, preterm delivery, and intrauterine growth retardation in pregnancies with nausea and vomiting (8,9).

There is no specific treatment for nausea and vomiting in pregnancy. However, there are practices that may help alleviate the symptoms (5,10–14). For example, small amounts of food should be consumed every 2 to 4 hours. An empty stomach may exacerbate the symptoms of nausea and vomiting, whereas eating large portions may increase gastric secretions and trigger nausea.

A small snack should be eaten before bedtime or during the night. This will help maintain normal glycemia throughout the night while preventing a drop in blood glucose levels during the early morning hours. An early morning snack, such as crackers or bread, can help raise the morning blood glucose level and prevent nausea. The woman can place the snack by the bed in the evening and consume it before getting out of bed in the morning. After eating the food, the woman should remain in bed for 30 minutes and then arise slowly, avoiding sudden movements.

Toothpaste can sometimes trigger nausea. It may help for women with morning sickness to avoid brushing their teeth immediately after eating or when they wake up. Substituting baking soda for toothpaste may also be advised.

As a general rule, liquids should be consumed 30 to 45 minutes after meals, or between meals. Caffeinated beverages, including coffee, tea, and chocolate, should be avoided because they could increase gastric secretions. Sugar-free carbonated beverages and carbonated water are recommended.

Fried, greasy, and high-fat foods, which can increase gastric acidity, should be avoided. Foods that are low in fat, such as lean meats, poultry without skin, and eggs, as well as easily digestible carbohydrate, may be better tolerated.

Cooking odors can exacerbate nausea and, if possible, should be avoided. Foods should be eaten cold or at room temperature. Ginger, which is used in teas and ginger ale and is available in powdered or capsule form, has been found to be effective in the treatment of nausea (15).

In women with GDM, nausea and vomiting can affect glycemic levels. In addition to following the previous recommendations, these women should eat a small amount (10 to 15 g) of carbohydrate every 2 to 3 hours to avoid low glycemic levels, and check urine ketones daily as long as they experience morning sickness. If necessary, the insulin therapy should be adjusted (16).

Hyperemesis Gravidarum

A more serious form of nausea and vomiting, hyperemesis gravidarum (HG), is associated with electrolyte imbalance, ketosis, dehydration, and weight loss (1,5,17). The symptoms of HG can compromise the health of the pregnant woman (jaundice, coma) and the fetus (preterm labor, low birth weight, intrauterine growth retardation) (3). Hyperemesis gravidarum occurs in approximately 2% to 3.5% of all pregnancies and may begin as early as the second month of gestation (1).

The exact cause of HG is unknown, but theories include thiamin deficiency, phosphate deficiency, hyperthyroidism, or psychological factors. Other conditions associated with severe nausea and vomiting, such as pancreatitis, cholecystitis, and thyroid disease, must be ruled out before a diagnosis of HG is made (8,18).

Management of HG focuses primarily on strategies that minimize nausea and vomiting and that reverse nutrient depletion (19). The course of treatment may include one or more of the following: traditional methods, enteral nutrition, medication, or parenteral nutrition.

In the traditional approach, the woman is admitted to the hospital and immediately given intravenous sodium chloride for rehydration (1). Solids may be reintroduced to the diet slowly, with clear liquids first, followed by a supplement and then soft, easily digestible solid foods. The patient is discharged when the vomiting ceases, when she can tolerate small frequent meals, and when it is evident that she is progressively gaining weight (19).

Very few studies of enteral feeding in the management of HG have been conducted (1). However, enteral nutrition may be a viable alternative if traditional treatment fails. Enteral feeding may be used once the woman is hydrated and her electrolytes are balanced (20).

The use of antiemetics in pregnancy is controversial because medications such as thalidomide have been associated with teratogenicity. Bendectin (doxylamine) was taken off the market in the United States, although no risks of birth defects were established; it is still available in Canada. Medications currently used for HG that have not been associated with teratogenic effects include chlorpromazine, phenothiazine, metoclopramide, prochlorperazine, pyridoxine, diphenhydramine, meclizine, and dimenhydrinate (3,11,12,21).

Parenteral nutrition is recommended for use in pregnancy only when the inability to tolerate enteral feeding threatens fetal health (1,8). Parenteral feeding can reverse the effects of weight loss and meet the nutritional requirements of the woman and fetus (22). Each individual must be carefully monitored to determine whether parenteral nutrition is indicated.

EXERCISE

Initial recommendations on exercise in pregnancy were published by the American College of Obstetricians and Gynecologists (ACOG) in 1994 (23). Women were instructed to limit exercise to less than 15 minutes, with target heart rates of fewer than 140 beats per minute. Exercise was thought to reduce oxygen flow to the placenta, resulting in fetal hypoxia or intrauterine growth retardation; however, this supposition was not based on clinical studies (24). ACOG has since revised its guidelines to reflect more recent research on the potential effects of exercise in pregnancy. Its current position is that women should continue to exercise during pregnancy if there are no medical or obstetric contraindications (25).

Effects on Pregnant Women and Fetuses

Maternal blood glucose is the main energy source for the fetus. Insulin sensitivity increases during exercise, which may increase the risk of hypoglycemia in the woman and limit the available glucose to the fetus (26). If the exposure to decreased maternal glucose is prolonged, ketosis could result and the fetus may be subject to malnutrition, intrauterine growth retardation, and low birth weight (24). Adequate energy intake is important in avoiding ketosis.

Exercise is associated with an increase in the pregnant woman's heat production and her metabolic rate (24,26). Teratogenic effects, particularly neural tube defects, are possible if the maternal temperature exceeds 37°C. This effect is not found in physically fit women, who may experience a reduction in their core temperature when they exercise. The decrease in temperature could reduce the effects of hyperthermic injury to the fetus (24,26).

Studies of the relationship between exercise and fetal growth have yielded conflicting results. Clapp et al found that the infants of women who exercised during pregnancy weighed less at birth than infants of women who did not exercise (27). However, Kardel and Kase found no such association (28). Clapp et al (29) tested the theory that exercise volume has no effect on fetal growth. The investigators found that a high volume of exercise performed at a moderate rate of intensity reduced infant birth weight. Conversely, a reduction in exercise volume increased the fat mass in the infant, but did not increase lean body mass (29).

Exercise during pregnancy may benefit women by reducing complications of labor and delivery, decreasing the pain and duration of labor, and promoting faster recovery after delivery. Other benefits include improved muscle tone, decreased nausea, fewer leg cramps, less lower back pain, fewer varicose veins, and less water retention (24–26,30). Exercise can strengthen abdominal and back muscles and improve coordination. It may also improve a woman's mental outlook and self-esteem (24,26).

Types, Duration, and Frequency of Exercise

Recommendations about exercise in pregnancy must be individualized. A woman's fitness level before she becomes pregnant, her current fitness level, and the week of gestation must be taken into consideration. It is necessary to instruct women about warning signs for complications. Pregnant women should stop exercising if they become excessively tired or overheated (24,25).

In most cases, women are able to engage in types of exercises that are similar to their prepregnancy exercise routines, although some adjustments to the duration, intensity, and frequency of exercise are usually made. Beginning a strenuous exercise routine in pregnancy, such as marathon running, is discouraged. Low-impact activities, such as walking, swimming, or using a stationary bicycle, are preferred. Women who were sedentary before pregnancy are encouraged to exercise, but they should be limited to low- to moderate-intensity activities. There are currently no exercise recommendations for the pregnant highly trained or elite athlete, although decreasing the intensity of the physical activity may prove beneficial.

Contact sports, such as hockey, soccer, volleyball, and basketball, increase the risk of trauma to the abdomen and should be avoided. Other high-risk activities, such as hang gliding, skydiving, or rock climbing, are discouraged. Gymnastics is considered unsafe in pregnancy because it involves sudden twists, turns, and bouncing. Experienced cross-country and downhill skiers may be able to continue skiing during the early part of their pregnancy, but they should not ski in late pregnancy. Any exercise that shifts the center of gravity, such as cycling, is not recommended. Exercises that compress the vena cava, such as those performed on the floor, are to be avoided after the first trimester (26). Scuba diving to depths below 30 feet is discouraged, because decompression may increase the risk of spontaneous abortion and preterm labor. Weight-bearing exercises should be limited to light weights. There are no studies to support or discourage the use of heavy weights in pregnancy.

The duration of exercise should not exceed 60 minutes, and pregnant women should not exercise to the point of exhaustion. The target heart rate in pregnancy is 140 beats per minute (bpm); however, 160 bpm may be acceptable for women who regularly exercised before they became pregnant (24).

Contraindications

Exercise is not recommended for all pregnant women. Contraindications to exercise in pregnancy include the following conditions: premature rupture of the membranes, preterm labor, incompetent cervix, cerclage, placenta previa, multiple gestation, preeclampsia or hypertension, anemia, intrauterine growth retardation, and any bleeding in the second or third trimesters. Pregnant women should seek prompt medical care if they experience contractions; pain in the chest, abdomen, or pelvic area; dizziness; or shortness of breath while exercising (24,26).

Pregnant women should not begin an exercise program until they have discussed the decision with their health care provider. Screening can rule out any medical or obstetric contraindications to exercising.

Recommendations and Guidelines for Women with Gestational Diabetes

There are no specific exercise recommendations for women with GDM. The 2004 position statement of the American Diabetes Association states, "Programs of moderate physical exercise have been shown to lower maternal glucose concentrations in women with GDM. Although the impact of exercise on neonatal complications awaits rigorous clinical trials, the beneficial glucose-lowering effects warrant a recommendation that women without medical or obstetrical contraindications be encouraged to start or continue a program of exercise as a part of treatment for GDM" (31). The summary statement of the Fourth International Workshop-Conference on Gestational Diabetes notes that exercise improves glucose tolerance and may obviate the need for insulin therapy (32).

Carpenter (33) found that exercise training augments medical nutrition therapy and improves birth outcome. The increased insulin sensitivity associated with increased physical activity can positively affect glucose levels in GDM (33). Bung et al (34) compared the efficacy of an exercise and diet regimen with the efficacy of diet and insulin therapy in 41 women with GDM for a 7- to 12-week period. There was no difference in the rate of complications between the two groups, including maternal hypoglycemia, fetal distress, infant birth weights or gestational age at delivery. The results of the study suggested that exercise is a viable option to insulin therapy in improving and maintaining glucose homeostasis in GDM (34). In a Brazilian study, researchers found a decrease in postprandial blood glucose levels when women with GDM participated in light exercise (walking) for 1 hour (35).

A study by Jovanovic-Peterson and Peterson evaluated the effects of five different exercises (stationary cycling, walking on a treadmill, rowing, recumbent cycling, and use of an upper-arm ergometer) on uterine activity (36). The researchers observed that the upper-arm ergometer was the safest form of exercise because it did not place stress on the lower body. The same upper-arm ergometer exercise regimen was then applied to 20 women with GDM randomized to two groups. One group was assigned to diet and exercise, (using the arm ergometer, three times a week, for 20 minutes at a time). The other group was assigned to intensive dietary therapy, but no exercise. After 6 weeks, the glycemic levels of the diet and exercise group were significantly improved compared with the diet-only group ($P < .001$).

A Canadian study examined the use of insulin in overweight women with GDM randomized into two groups, diet and resistance training vs diet alone. The women in the diet and exercise group had a lower incidence of insulin treatment and delayed insulin initiation than women in the diet-only group (37).

A program for women with GDM advises women to rest and monitor fetal activity before and immediately after exercise (38). The duration of the exercise is limited to 30 minutes after eating. Women are instructed to refrain from exercising if their blood glucose level is less than 60 mg/dL or more than 250 mg/dL, or if there are fewer than ten fetal movements in a 24-hour period (38). A summary of guidelines and contraindications of exercise in pregnancy is found in Box 8.1 (23–26,39,40).

Adequate hydration is important during and after the exercise (26). The amount of fluid lost in exercise is determined by monitoring weight before and after exercising. A

BOX 8.1

Guidelines and Contraindications for Exercise in GDM

GUIDELINES

- Exercise 1 to 2 hours after a meal. Do not exercise before eating.
- Monitor blood glucose level before exercising.
- Do not exercise during peak insulin action times.
- If necessary to keep blood glucose in target range, eat a snack before exercising.
- Avoid injecting insulin into areas of the body that will be used during exercising.
- Maternal heart rate should not exceed 140 beats per minute.
- Maternal blood pressure should not exceed 149/90 mm Hg.
- Limit exercise to light- or moderate-intensity activities.
- Consume sufficient fluids to stay hydrated. Adequate fluid intake is important to avoid dehydration and possible preterm labor.
- Consume sufficient energy to avoid hypoglycemia and ketosis.
- Do not exercise in hot or humid weather.

CONTRAINDICATIONS

- Pregnancy-induced hypertension or preeclampsia
- Premature rupture of membranes
- Preterm labor
- Incompetent cervix or cerclage
- Persistent bleeding in the second or third trimester
- Indications of intrauterine growth retardation
- Blood glucose levels <60 mg/dL or >250 mg/dL
- Presence of ketonuria
- Multiple gestations
- History of three or more spontaneous abortions
- Morbid obesity

Source: Data are from references 23–26 and 39–40.

weight loss of 1 lb during activity equals 16 oz of fluid. Any fluid loss should be replaced before the next exercise session (30). Exercising in hot or humid weather is not recommended.

ADOLESCENTS WITH GDM

In the United States, children comprise 19% of the population (41). Fifteen million US children live in poverty (41). The importance of promoting preventive health care for adolescents cannot be overemphasized.

The prevalence of GDM in adolescents is unknown. At present, there is no specific medical nutrition therapy protocol specifically designed for the adolescent with GDM.

Torres et al analyzed serum glucose concentrations to study GDM and glucose intolerance in 115 pregnant Mexicans younger than 18 years (42). A 1-hour, 50-g glucose challenge test (GCT) was performed at 24 to 28 (n = 103) or at 29 to 35 (n = 12) weeks' gestation, and an oral glucose tolerance test (OGTT) was administered 3 to 5 days later. Eight subjects had abnormal GCTs, and three of these individuals had abnormal OGTTs. Sixteen adolescents (13 with previously normal GCT) had abnormal OGTTs; 15 of these girls were classified as having gestational glucose intolerance (GGI), and one was diagnosed with GDM. The study reported that the serum glucose concentration in pregnant women younger than 25 years during an OGTT was lower than in their older counterparts. Serum glucose concentrations in adolescents with GGI were higher than in adolescents with normal OGTT at 60 and 120 minutes during the OGTT ($P < .001$) and when expressed as the area under the glucose curve ($P < .001$). Adolescents with GGI had serum glucose concentrations during the OGTT similar to adult, nondiabetic, pregnant Mexican women. The authors suggested that GGI in pregnant adolescents may represent an early sign that glucose metabolism will deteriorate in the future. GGI may lead to a higher risk of GDM in future pregnancies and/or type 2 diabetes in adulthood. The authors concluded that the current criteria used to diagnose GDM in adults may not entirely apply to adolescents (42). This may be especially true in ethnic groups at high risk for glucose abnormalities or when there is a frequency of multiparous adolescents, as seen in developing countries.

It is not clear whether it is cost effective to screen all pregnant adolescents for GDM. A study was conducted to identify the prevalence of GDM in a group of 632 adolescents and to examine the risk factors that identify those at greatest risk for developing GDM (43). Eleven of the adolescents developed GDM, and a higher prevalence of GDM was found in adolescents whose body mass index (BMI) was greater than 27 ($P < .001$). BMI is an important risk factor in the development of GDM in adolescents. The authors recommended selective screening for GDM in adolescents based on their prepregnancy BMI.

A retrospective review of 326 women younger than 20 years, who identified themselves as Hispanic American, was conducted to determine the incidence of GDM in Hispanic adolescents (44). Thirty subjects (9.2%) had abnormal glucose levels (≥ 140 mg/dL) after the GCT. Five were diagnosed with GDM after the OGTT was administered. The incidence of GDM was 1.5% (5/326) (95% CI, 0.6–3.7). The researchers concluded that the incidence of GDM in adolescent Hispanic Americans is so low that universal screening may not be warranted.

The lack of research about GDM in adolescents is alarming, in view of the high rates of obesity and diabetes in this population. There is no consensus at present as to whether universal screening for GDM should be recommended for pregnant adolescents or whether the test should be different from the test used to diagnose GDM in adult women. This is an open field for additional scientific research.

SUBSTANCE ABUSE

The use of legal or illegal substances, such as alcohol, tobacco, cocaine, heroin, and marijuana, during pregnancy may have a devastating effect on perinatal outcome. Maternal substance use is associated with preterm delivery, low birth weight, and congenital anomalies (45). The effects can range from temporary (withdrawal symptoms in the newborn exposed to heroin in utero) to permanent (fetal alcohol syndrome). If a woman uses more than one substance, that can make it difficult to evaluate the consequences for the fetus. Also, other problems, such as low incomes, inadequate prenatal care, and poor nutrition, may complicate pregnancy in women who use illicit substances.

A literature search found no studies that specifically address substance abuse and GDM. However, understanding the key effects and treatment modalities can help practitioners to provide the prenatal care and educational services needed by women with GDM.

Alcohol

Alcohol is a legal substance, but it is also a leading cause of infant morbidity and mortality in the United States (46). Alcohol use in pregnancy may cause fetal alcohol syndrome, which is characterized by growth and mental retardation, facial dysmorphologies, and central nervous system abnormalities (45,47). Other fetal effects associated with alcohol use in pregnancy include hyperactivity and low intelligence quotients (45,48). In the pregnant woman, alcohol use may increase the risk of placental abruption, preterm delivery, and spontaneous abortion (49).

No safe level of alcohol in pregnancy has been determined. The US Surgeon General recommends that all women abstain from alcohol during pregnancy (50). Although the most critical time in pregnancy is the first 56 days after conception (the organogenesis period), when the major fetal structures are developing, the effect of alcohol on the fetus is not limited to the first trimester. Alcohol can harm the fetus throughout pregnancy, and the neonate may experience withdrawal symptoms immediately after birth (45,47,49).

Alcohol can also have an effect on the pregnant woman's nutritional status by interfering with the storage and utilization of nutrients. It impairs the absorption of nutrients and alters their transport for metabolic use (51). If calories from alcohol (7 kcal/g) replace food calories in the diet, the result may be malnutrition (52). Alcohol may also affect the blood glucose level. Alcohol inhibits hepatic gluconeogenesis, increasing the risk of hypoglycemia especially if alcohol replaces food (53).

In a large retrospective cohort study, GDM was found to occur less often in women who drank alcohol (54). However, even if alcohol has a protective effect against GDM, the adverse effects to the fetus would not warrant the consumption of alcohol during pregnancy.

Tobacco

No congenital anomalies have been associated with smoking, but a higher incidence of low birth weight, intrauterine growth retardation, and sudden infant death syndrome is associated with cigarette smoking in pregnant women (48). Preterm delivery, premature rupture of the membranes, placenta previa, spontaneous abortion, and placental abruption are all associated with tobacco use in pregnant women (45). The nutritional risks to the pregnant woman who smokes include inadequate nutrient stores resulting from a poor intake. Women who give up smoking while pregnant may experience strong cravings for refined carbohydrates, which may lead to excessive weight gain and higher blood glucose level (55).

Cocaine

Cocaine, especially in the form of crack, is a highly addictive drug. The effect of cocaine on the central nervous system is rapid, giving the user a quick feeling of euphoria. Cocaine is a powerful vasoconstrictor, which can lead to hypertension, stroke, or sudden death. If a pregnant woman uses cocaine, the fetus is at increased risk of intrauterine growth retardation and fetal demise caused by a reduction in oxygen and nutrient supply. Infants whose mothers are addicted to cocaine may experience jitteriness, seizures, and frantic sucking reflexes (55,56). They are also at risk of developing neurobehavioral difficulties (55).

Pregnant women who use cocaine have an increased risk of preterm delivery, premature rupture of the membranes, placental abruption, preeclampsia, and spontaneous abortion

(45). The nutritional effects associated with cocaine use are decreased appetite, altered taste perception, constipation, and weight loss (57). Cocaine can also increase the breakdown of glycogen and can raise the blood glucose level (58).

Heroin

Heroin and other opiates can have a devastating effect on women and fetuses. Heroin use in pregnant women is associated with a higher rate of spontaneous abortion, intrauterine growth retardation, preterm delivery, and fetal demise (45,56). Infants whose mothers use heroin during pregnancy are at increased risk of jaundice, low birth weight, and seizures, and they may experience withdrawal symptoms (56). They are poor feeders and may experience vomiting, diarrhea, and weight loss. The woman is at risk for anemia and pregnancy-induced hypertension. The perinatal outcome may be improved if the pregnant woman undergoes methadone treatment (45). During detoxification, the woman may suffer from constipation, nausea, vomiting, or inadequate dietary intake, which may affect the blood glucose level (58).

Marijuana

Marijuana use is associated with tachycardia, bronchitis, sinusitis, and pharyngitis (45). Its use in pregnancy has not been associated with any teratogenic effects to the fetus. Low birth weight has been associated with marijuana use (45). Maternal effects may include higher-than-normal risks of spontaneous abortion and poor weight gain (45). Marijuana use can also increase appetite, which causes overeating that can lead to hyperglycemia (58).

Hallucinogens

There are no known effects of hallucinogens, such as LSD, acid, or ecstasy, on pregnancy. However, the adverse effects of these drugs include dizziness, weakness, nausea, and panic attacks (45,59). No withdrawal symptoms have been associated with this class of drugs. Additional studies are needed to determine the long-term effect of hallucinogens on the infant.

Medical Nutrition Therapy in Substance Abuse Treatment

Pregnant substance-abusing women may have long-standing nutritional disorders caused by irregular or poor eating habits and inadequate dietary intake. According to the position statement of the American Dietetic Association on nutrition intervention and chemical dependency, "Nutrition intervention, planned and provided by a qualified nutrition professional, is an essential component of the treatment and recovery from chemical dependency" (60).

Malnutrition can be a major complication in the substance-abusing individual. A meal plan that is low in fat and includes adequate protein, complex carbohydrates, and fiber can combat the effects of prolonged poor eating habits. Regular mealtimes are important for individuals in drug rehabilitation. A multivitamin-mineral supplement may be used to replenish nutrient deficiencies. Dehydration is common, and an adequate fluid intake must be emphasized (51,60). There is a risk that individuals may overeat, replacing one addiction with another.

SUMMARY

Complications unique to pregnancy can affect maternal glycemic levels and the pregnancy outcome in various ways. Certain conditions, such as nausea and vomiting, are often unavoidable but can be made tolerable with nutrition management. If there are no contraindications, exercise may have a beneficial effect on glycemic levels in women with GDM. Pregnant adolescents with GDM require special attention to maintain optimal glucose control and to provide adequate nutrients for maternal and fetal growth. Substance abuse in pregnancy may have a detrimental effect on the health of the woman and the fetus.

REFERENCES

1. American College of Obstetricians and Gynecologists. ACOG (American College of Obstetrics and Gynecology) Practice Bulletin. Nausea and vomiting in pregnancy. *Obstet Gynecol.* 2004; 103:803–814.
2. Scott LD, Abu-Hamda E. Gastrointestinal disease in pregnancy. In: Creasy R, Resnik R, Iams JD, eds. *Maternal-Fetal Medicine: Principles and Practices.* 5th ed. Philadelphia, Pa: Elsevier; 2004:1109–1125.
3. Quinla JD, Hill DA. Nausea and vomiting of pregnancy. *Am Fam Physician.* 2003;68:121–128.
4. Gadsby R, Barnie-Adshead AM, Jagger C. A prospective study of nausea and vomiting during pregnancy. *Br J Gen Pract.* 1993;43:245–248.
5. Koch KL, Frissora CL. Nausea and vomiting during pregnancy. *Gastroenterol Clin North Am.* 2003;32:201–234.
6. Soules MR, Hughes CL Jr, Garcia JA, Livengood CH, Prystowsky MR, Alexander E. Nausea and vomiting of pregnancy: role of human chorionic gonadotropin and 17-hydroxyprogesterone. *Obstet Gynecol.* 1980;55:696–700.
7. Goodwin TM. Nausea and vomiting of pregnancy: an obstetric syndrome. *Am J Obstet Gynecol.* 2002;186(Suppl 5):S184-S189.
8. Hill WC, Fleming AD. Gastrointestinal diseases complicating pregnancy. In: Reece EA, Hobbins JC, eds. *Medicine of the Fetus and the Mother.* Philadelphia, Pa: Lippincott-Raven; 1999:1123–1152.
9. Weigel MM, Weigel RM. Nausea and vomiting of early pregnancy and pregnancy outcome. An epidemiological study. *Br J Obstet Gynaecol.* 1989;96:1304–1311.
10. Erick E. *No More Morning Sickness.* New York, NY: Penguin Books; 1993.
11. Niebyl JR, Goodwin TM. Overview of nausea and vomiting of pregnancy with an emphasis on vitamins and ginger. *Am J Obstet Gynecol.* 2002;186(Suppl 5):S253-S255.
12. Magee LA, Mazzota P, Koren G. Evidence-based view of safety and effectiveness of pharmacologic therapy for nausea and vomiting of pregnancy (NVP). *Am J Obstet Gynecol.* 2002;186(Suppl 5): S256-S61.
13. Portnoi G, Chung LA, Karimi-Tabesh L, Koren G, Tan MP, Einarson A. Prospective comparative study of the safety and effectiveness of ginger for the treatment of nausea and vomiting in pregnancy. *Am J Obstet Gynecol.* 2003;189:1374–1377.
14. Smith C, Crowther C, Willson K, Hotham N, McMillian V. A randomized controlled trial of ginger to treat nausea and vomiting in pregnancy. *Obstet Gynecol.* 2004;103:639–645.
15. Fischer-Rasmussen W, Kjaer SK, Dahl C, Asping U. Ginger treatment of hyperemesis gravidarum. *Eur J Obstet Gynecol Reprod Biol.* 1991;38:19–24.
16. *American Dietetic Association Medical Nutrition Therapy Evidence-Based Guides for Practice: Nutrition Practice Guidelines for Gestational Diabetes Mellitus* [CD-ROM]. Chicago, Ill: American Dietetic Association; 2001.
17. Furneaux EC, Langley-Evans AJ, Langley-Evans SC. Nausea and vomiting of pregnancy: endocrine basis and contribution to pregnancy outcome. *Obstet Gynecol Surv.* 2001;56:775–782.
18. Crump WJ, Aten LA. Hyperemesis, hyperthyroidism or both? *J Fam Pract.* 1992;34:450, 453–456.

19. Rodwell Williams S, Trahms CM. Management of pregnancy complications and special maternal disease conditions. In: Worthington-Roberts BS, Rodwell Williams S, eds. *Nutrition in Pregnancy and Lactation*. 6th ed. Dubuque, Iowa: Brown and Benchmark; 1997:254–291.

20. Barclay BA. Experience with enteral nutrition in the treatment of hyperemesis gravidarum. *Nutr Clin Pract*. 1990;5:153–155.

21. Gordon MC. Maternal physiology in pregnancy. In: Gabbe SG, Niebyl JR, Simpson JL. *Obstetrics: Normal and Problem Pregnancies*. Philadelphia, Pa: Churchill Livingstone; 2002:63–91.

22. Zibell-Frisk D, Jen KLC, Rick J. Use of parenteral nutrition to maintain adequate nutritional status in hyperemesis gravidarum. *J Perinatol*. 1990;10:390–395.

23. Exercise during pregnancy and the postpartum period. ACOG Technical Bulletin Number 189—February 1994. *Int J Gynaecol Obstet*. 1994;45:65–70.

24. Smith CS, Van Andel R. Pregnancy and North American lifestyles: exercise, work and diet in pregnancy. *Clin Fam Pract*. 2001;3:167–181.

25. ACOG Committee Obstetric Practice. ACOG Committee opinion. Number 267, January 2002: exercise during pregnancy and the postpartum period. *Obstet Gynecol*. 2002;99:171–173.

26. Carlson B, Parrish D. Exercising During Pregnancy: What to Tell Your Patients. Available at: http://www.womenshealthpc.com/3_98/pdf/171ExercisePregnancy3_98.pdf. Accessed December 7, 2004.

27. Clapp JF 3rd, Simonian S, Lopez B, Appleby-Wineberg S, Harcar-Sevcik R. The one-year morphometric and neurodevelopmental outcome of the offspring of women who continued to exercise regularly throughout pregnancy. *Am J Obstet Gynecol*. 1998;178:594–599.

28. Kardel KR, Kase T. Training in pregnant women: effects on fetal development and birth. *Am J Obstet Gynecol*. 1998;178:280–286.

29. Clapp JF, Kim H, Burciu B, Schmidt S, Petry K, Lopez B. Continuing regular exercise during pregnancy: effect of exercise volume on fetoplacental growth. *Am J Obstet Gynecol*. 2002;186:142–147.

30. Artal R, O'Toole M. Guidelines of the American College of Obstetricians and Gynecologists for exercise during pregnancy and the postpartum period. *Br J Sports Med*. 2003;37:6–12.

31. American Diabetes Association. Gestational diabetes mellitus. *Diabetes Care*. 2004;27(Suppl 1):S88-S90.

32. Jovanovic L. American Diabetes Association's Fourth International Workshop-Conference on Gestational Diabetes Mellitus: summary and discussion. Therapeutic interventions. *Diabetes Care*. 1998;21(Suppl 2):B131-B137.

33. Carpenter MW. The role of exercise in pregnant women with diabetes mellitus. *Clin Obstet Gynecol*. 2000;43:56–64.

34. Bung P, Artal R, Khodiguian N, Kjos S. Exercise in gestational diabetes. An optional therapeutic approach? *Diabetes*. 1991;40(Suppl 2):S182-S185.

35. Garcia-Patterson A, Martin E, Ubeda J, Maria MA, de Leiva A, Corcoy R. Evaluation of light exercise in the treatment of gestational diabetes. *Diabetes Care*. 2001;24:2006–2007.

36. Jovanovic-Peterson L, Peterson CM. Is exercise safe or useful for gestational diabetic women? *Diabetes*. 1991;40(Suppl 2):S179-S181.

37. Brankston GN, Mitchell BF, Ryan EA, Okun NB. Resistance exercise decreases the need for insulin in overweight women with gestational diabetes mellitus. *Am J Obstet Gynecol*. 2004;190:188–193.

38. Artal R, Masaki DI. Exercise in gestational diabetes. A new therapeutic approach. *Pract Diabetol*. 1989;8:7014.

39. Holler HJ, Green Pastors J. *Diabetes Medical Nutrition Therapy*. Chicago, Ill: American Dietetic Association; 1997.

40. Artal R. Exercise: the alternative therapeutic intervention for gestational diabetes. *Clin Obstet Gynecol*. 2003;46:479–487.

41. Clayton S, Brindis C, Hamor J, Raiden-Wright H, Fong C. Investing in adolescent health. A social imperative for California's future. National Adolescent Health Information Center, University of California, San Francisco. Available at: http://www.mch.dhs.ca.gov/documents/pdf/caadolhlthcollabstraegicplan.pdf. Accessed December 7, 2004.

42. Ramirez-Torres MA, Rodriguez-Pezino J, Zambrana-Castenda M, Lira-Plascencia J, Parra A. Gestational diabetes mellitus and glucose intolerance among Mexican pregnant adolescents. *J Pediatr Endocrinol Metab.* 2003;163:401–405.

43. Khine ML, Winklestein K, Copel JA. Selective screening for gestational diabetes mellitus in adolescent pregnancies. *Obstet Gynecol.* 1999;93:738–742.

44. Southwick RD, Wigton TR. Screening for gestational diabetes mellitus in adolescent Hispanic Americans. *J Reprod Med.* 2000;45:31–34.

45. American College of Obstetricians and Gynecologists. Substance abuse in pregnancy. ACOG Technical Bulletin Number 195—July 1994 (replaces No. 96, September 1986). *Int J Gynaecol Obstet.* 1994;47:73–80.

46. Svikis DS, Reid-Quinones K. Screening and prevention of alcohol and drug use disorders in women. *Obstet Gynecol Clin North Am.* 2003;30:447–468.

47. Bolnick JM, Rayburn WF. Substance use disorders in women: special considerations during pregnancy. *Obstet Gynecol Clin North Am.* 2003;30:545–558.

48. Streissguth AP, Sampson PD, Barr HM, Bookstein FL, Carmichael Olson H. The effects of prenatal exposure to alcohol and tobacco. Contributions from the Seattle longitudinal prospective study and implications for public policy. In: Needleman HL, Bellinger D. *Prenatal Exposure to Toxicants.* Baltimore, Md: John Hopkins University Press; 1994:148–183.

49. Streissguth AP. *Fetal Alcohol Syndrome. A Guide for Families and Communities.* Baltimore, Md: Paul H Brooks Publishing; 1997.

50. US Department of Health and Human Services. Surgeon General's advisory on alcohol and pregnancy. *FDA Drug Bull.* 1981;11:9–10.

51. National Institute on Alcohol Abuse and Alcoholism. Alcohol Alert. 1993;22:PH346. Available at: http://www.niaaa.nih.gov/publications/aa22.htm. Accessed December 7, 2004.

52. Feinman L, Lieber CS. Nutrition. In: Miller NS, ed. *Principles of Addiction Medicine.* Chevy Chase, Md: American Society of Addiction Medicine; 1994:741–753.

53. Nelson PA, Kilbury A. Nutritional support of pregnant diabetic patients. In: Nuwayhid BS, Brinkman CR, Lieb SM, eds. *Management of the Diabetic Pregnancy.* New York, NY: Elsevier; 1987:168–213.

54. Xiong X, Saunders LD, Wang FL, Demianczuk NN. Gestational diabetes mellitus: prevalence, risk factors, maternal and infant outcomes. *Int J Gynaecol Obstet.* 2001;75:221–228.

55. Russell CA. Addiction, nutrition and health. *Dent Health (London).* 1985;24:7, 9–11.

56. Day NL, Richardson GA, McGauhey PJ. The effects of prenatal exposure to marijuana, cocaine, heroin and methadone. In: Needleman HL, Bellinger D. *Prenatal Exposure to Toxicants.* Baltimore, Md: Johns Hopkins University Press; 1994:184–209.

57. National Institutes of Health. Diet and substance abuse recovery. Available at: http://www.nlm.nih.gov/medlineplus/ency/article/002149.htm. Accessed December 7, 2004.

58. Glick D. Before you party: are you in the danger zone? *Diabetes Interview.* 2003;12;57.

59. Witter FR. Principles of tetratology of drugs and radiation. In: Winn HN, Hobbins JC, eds. *Clinical Maternal-Fetal Medicine.* New York, NY: Parthenon Publishing Group; 2000:813–815.

60. American Dietetic Association. Position of the American Dietetic Association: nutrition intervention in treatment and recovery from chemical dependency. *J Am Diet Assoc.* 1990;90:1274–1277.

9

Cultural Issues in Diabetes Management in Pregnancy

Yolanda M. Gutierrez, MS, PhD, RD

OBJECTIVES   After completing this chapter, you will be able to do the following:

1. Summarize the incidence of gestational diabetes mellitus (GDM) nationally and globally.
2. Identify the cultural and ethnic issues that influence patient care.
3. Discuss issues and themes that guide the development of GDM care and education.

BACKGROUND

Pregnancy is a time of physical and emotional changes for all women. For pregnant women with GDM, concerns about having a normal, healthy child and/or neonatal morbidity are magnified. When a woman learns that she has developed GDM, she faces increased responsibilities for fetal development and diabetes management. A woman's reaction to the diagnosis will be shaped by several factors, including her established habits and family/cultural patterns for managing health, as well as her personality and learned coping methods. This chapter presents an overview of the incidence of and genetic predisposition for GDM. It also discusses how ethnicity and culture affect diabetes care and the demands on the health care team.

PREVALENCE OF GDM IN RACIAL AND ETHNIC GROUPS

The prevalence of GDM varies markedly among racial and ethnic groups, among regions of the country, and in different parts of the world (1). O'Sullivan and Mahan (2) reported a GDM prevalence of 2.6% in Boston, whereas Mestman (3) reported a prevalence of 12.3% in Los Angeles. According to Mestman (3), this difference in the prevalence between the two cities can be explained by the number of obese Hispanic women (Mexican Americans) in the Los Angeles area. In Australia, the prevalence of GDM differs according to country of birth, ranging from 4.3% for women born in Australia and New Zealand to 15% for women born on the Indian subcontinent (4).

The reported prevalence of GDM can vary depending on the testing methods and diagnostic criteria used. In North America, the National Diabetes Data Group (NDDG) (5) recommends a definition of GDM based on data from O'Sullivan and Mahan (2). Other countries, however, use different diagnostic criteria, from the World Health Organization (WHO) (6). As a result, it can be difficult to compare statistics for the United States with those from other nations. (For more information on diagnosis of GDM and maternal testing, see Chapters 3 and 5.)

GENETIC PREDISPOSITION FOR GDM

Although there are few studies that focus on the issue of genetic predisposition in GDM, diabetes educators and dietetics professionals may find insights in studies that evaluate culture, genetics, and the incidence of type 1 and type 2 diabetes.

The genetics of diabetes is complex, and it is unlikely that a single major gene accounts for a substantial proportion of occurrence of the disease. Unique genetic markers, however, have become important in admixture studies, which investigate the role genetics plays in the association between race or ethnicity and disease (7–10). For example, insulin resistance and acute insulin response were shown to vary as a function of genetic markers that act as surrogates for proportions of African ancestry (8). The admixture approach has also been used in the study of type 2 diabetes in Pima Indians (9) and type 1 diabetes in African Americans (10). The findings from these studies suggest that there are genetic differences across races and ethnicities, but extreme caution is required when interpreting the results.

FAMILY HISTORY AND PREDISPOSITION FOR GDM

Information on family history may serve as a useful tool for public health and preventive medicine. Family history reflects both genetic and environmental factors and may serve as a better predictor of diabetes risk than either type of factor alone. The San Antonio Heart Study, for example, examined a large population sample of Mexican Americans and non-Hispanic whites. Analyses stratified by gender and adjusted for age and ethnicity showed that men with diabetes were more than three times as likely to have one or both parents with diabetes; whereas for women, only the maternal history was significantly associated with diabetes (11).

CULTURAL AND ETHNIC ISSUES THAT INFLUENCE PATIENT CARE

Because ethnicity and culture influence how people think, feel, and behave, these factors play a key role in determining how individuals experience life: what to eat; how to work, play, raise children, and celebrate holidays; and the experience of pregnancy, illness, and death (12,13). Cultural differences between health professionals and clients can create stress and can affect patient care. For example, a pregnant woman may be coping with the stress of emigration and acculturation, and her first priority may be her day-to-day survival. Issues of acculturation and the length of time the individual has lived in the United States can have a powerful impact on her food choices, food availability, and her beliefs about food and illness (12,13). The customs and folk beliefs of the individual can also have consequences for patient care. In many cultures, pregnant women fear the interference of evil spirits in the process of pregnancy and birth (12,13).

Culturally appropriate nutrition assessment and interventions for high-risk populations must take into account cultural variations in disease susceptibility, health care access, disease definition, risk estimation, and lifestyle behaviors (14,15). A study that evaluated family history data collection among Pacific Islanders living in the United States found that subjects did not always report diabetes in family members (14). In a study undertaken as part of the Alliance of Black Churches Health Project, rural African Americans who defined diabetes as "sugar" or "sugar-diabetes" believed their condition was less serious, and had higher glucose levels, than those who defined their disease as diabetes (16).

The increasing diversity of the US population, changes in health care, and the epidemic of obesity in the nation have prompted the government and other organizations to expand their collection of health education materials and professional resources. These include reproductive, maternal, and child health materials available in English, Spanish, and some Asian languages, such as Chinese and Vietnamese.

CULTURAL COMPETENCY

To prepare themselves to effectively work with individuals from different ethnic or racial origins, health care providers should understand the meaning of the terms "cultural competency" and "cultural sensitivity." The Health Resources and Services Administration Bureau of Health Professions, Division of Nursing defines *cultural competency* as a set of academic and interpersonal skills that allow individuals to increase their understanding and appreciation of cultural differences and similarities within, among, and between groups (17).

Cultural sensitivity is an awareness of one's own cultural beliefs, assumptions, customs, and values, as well as those of other cultural groups. Cultural sensitivity in counseling requires a special effort that excludes personal bias in making value judgments about people from other racial or ethnic groups (13).

Health care practitioners must be culturally competent to be effective. Regardless of their ethnic, racial, cultural, socioeconomic, and educational backgrounds, all patients recognize when they are treated with respect. The Cultural Competence Works Report identifies the following stages in learning to become culturally competent (18):

1. *Cultural awareness*—the process of self-assessment. The individual examines his or her own learned biases and prejudices toward other cultures while making an effort to become sensitive to another person's values, beliefs, lifestyles, and problem-solving strategies.
2. *Cultural knowledge*—the process of learning about the world views of other cultures. This is usually accomplished through books, workshops, self-study, audiovisual presentations, and other classroom techniques.
3. *Cultural skill.* Cultural skill develops as practitioners learn to assess relevant factors related to the client that will affect nutrition education.

To become culturally competent, health care providers must be aware of many different aspects of culture, including the following:

- *Time*. People from different cultures may schedule their time differently. For example, whites may fill up their appointment books many months in advance, whereas many Latinos schedule appointments as the need arises.

- *Decision making.* For example, in many cultures (eg, Hispanics, Native Indians, Southeast Asians), the husband is the primary decision maker on what to eat, what to buy, and the course of treatment if his wife requires insulin.
- *Causes of illness.* In some situations, a husband may blame his wife for developing diabetes and he may conclude that if his wife consumes only a small amount of food, her blood glucose level will improve. However, a restricted diet could result in inadequate energy intake and weight loss. A culturally sensitive health care provider will ask questions, listen attentively, and avoid making assumptions that everything is fine just because the woman's blood glucose level is normal. Thus, cultural sensitivity allows the practitioner to intervene on the woman's behalf.
- *Support.* The health care provider needs to ask whether the woman has a support system, lives alone, or has family in the United States. These issues will influence the management and treatment of the woman's diabetes.
- *Food.* The woman must understand that she does not have to purchase special foods because she has diabetes. This is a very common myth. The health care provider must determine what, why, when, and how much the woman eats. The practitioner should also teach the client how to properly distribute carbohydrate throughout the day and how to meet her nutrient needs as well as those of the fetus. (For more information regarding maternal nutrient needs, see Chapter 6.)

The LEARN Approach

The LEARN (*L*isten, *E*xplain, *A*cknowledge, *R*ecommend, *N*egotiate) approach is an effective model for working with people from different cultures (19,20). This approach emphasizes the responsibility of health care professionals to learn from their clients. When working with women with GDM, practitioners need to determine what role the client feels she has in caring for her pregnancy and learn what beliefs she has about treatments for diabetes. Once the patient's beliefs are acknowledged and appreciated, the interdisciplinary health care team can then recommend medical and psychosocial guidelines and negotiate the components of the care plan that may be perceived as threatening or opposed to the woman's values or beliefs.

When recommending specific meal plans for women with GDM, diabetes educators and dietetics professionals should understand that compliance with dietary advice may be poor for cultural reasons. For example, a woman with GDM may find it impractical to modify the diet of her entire family, despite the dietetics professional's explanation that "the diabetic diet" is healthy and advisable for all family members. Other cultural reasons for noncompliance are that some cultures equate obesity with health and prosperity and that most cultures do not measure the amount of food eaten. For example, in Hispanic culture, people do not learn to cook by following recipes or measuring ingredients.

Strategies for improving compliance include enlisting the expertise of dietetics professionals who are knowledgeable about the woman's culture and have the necessary linguistic skills and the ability to adapt their teaching styles to the individual client. Health care teams that do not have access to this expertise may consider using diet sheets and other teaching aids. The American Dietetic Association (ADA) has a series of booklets on ethnic and regional food practices, with diabetes food guide pyramids in several languages. See ADA's Web site (21) for further information.

HEALTH CARE PROVIDERS' RESPONSIBILITIES ACROSS DISCIPLINES

It is critical that all members of the health care team agree on the principles of care for women with GDM and understand cultural issues that are involved in the delivery of that care. The following sections identify responsibilities that members of the health care team share.

Nutrition Education

The entire interdisciplinary health care team is responsible for educating clients about healthful dietary choices. The recommended diet should do the following:

- Meet the individual's requirements for essential nutrients
- Minimize the risk of chronic diseases
- Avoid excesses
- Be safe from toxins
- Be culturally acceptable
- Be affordable
- Be palatable and readily available

When a woman with GDM and her family learn fundamental nutrition principles, her compliance with diabetes medical nutrition therapy is likely to improve. The following are key points that dietetics professionals should cover in counseling sessions with women with GDM:

- *Hydration.* Dietetics professionals should stress the importance of getting enough fluids. According to the 2005 Dietary Guidelines for Americans, normal drinking behavior (ie, drinking when thirsty and having fluids with meals) is usually sufficient (22). See Chapter 8 for hydration guidelines for exercise.
- *Eating regular meals and snacks.* Dietetics professionals should encourage regular meals (three meals and two to three snacks every day). Emphasis should be placed on healthful drinks and snacks, including nonfat milk, fresh fruit, low-fat yogurt, celery, and peanut butter.
- *Avoiding fast food and controlling portion sizes.* The woman with GDM should avoid fast foods and be careful with portion sizes (avoiding "large," "big," and "deluxe" menu options).
- *Physical activity.* Dietetics professionals should encourage physical activity (see Chapter 8).
- *Self-esteem.* Whenever possible, dietetics professionals should give messages of self-acceptance to improve self-esteem.

Learning From Cultural Competence Publications

Using cultural competence to improve the quality of health care for diverse populations adds value to managed care arrangements. The interdisciplinary health care team should regularly refer to cultural competence publications for guidance in treating diverse populations. A list of publications can be found in the Cultural Competence Works report at HRSA's Web site (18).

Acting as a Cultural Broker as Well as an Advocate

Melville defines "cultural brokers" as individuals who guide and teach others issues related to their culture (23) (eg, holidays, special beliefs, or values about food). An example of a cultural broker is the child born in the United States whose parents were born in another country. When the child goes to school and learns American customs and festivities, he or she becomes a cultural broker by teaching the parents about Thanksgiving and other holiday traditions. For the health care professional, being a cultural broker means teaching clients from different cultures how to make healthful food choices in the United States—eg, opting for salads instead of high-fat fast foods.

Referrals and Follow-Up Appointments

Women with GDM may seek health care in settings that do not include all health disciplines, and in these situations referrals to outside experts can be crucial. For example, if dietetics professionals are not associated with a clinic or office, women with GDM should be referred to a dietitian with expertise in diabetes and pregnancy. If women experience symptoms of depression, they should be referred to a social worker or therapist.

Health care professionals also need to help clients to schedule and remember follow-up appointments.

SUMMARY

In working with a diverse population, cultural competence is important in the care of the GDM patient. When working with people from different cultures, the health care team can use the LEARN Approach- Listen, Explain, Acknowledge, Recommend, and Negotiate.

Nutrition counseling is a cornerstone in the management of women with diabetes from diverse cultural or ethnic groups. All women with GDM, regardless of their backgrounds, must receive medical nutrition therapy to promote normoglycemia, to avoid excessive or insufficient weight gain, and to meet their nutrient requirements. The health care team has important responsibilities to ensure that these goals are achieved. These responsibilities include standardizing nutrition information, teaching fundamental nutrition concepts, improving the client's dietary habits, keeping abreast of current nutrition research, and, when necessary, referring the patient to other health care professionals with expertise in diabetes and pregnancy.

REFERENCES

1. American Diabetes Association. Gestational diabetes. In: *Medical Management of Pregnancy Complicated by Diabetes*. 3rd ed. Alexandria, Va: American Diabetes Association. 2000:114–132.
2. O'Sullivan JB, Mahan CM. Criteria for the oral glucose tolerance test in pregnancy. *Diabetes*. 1964;13:278–285.
3. Mestman JH. Outcome of diabetes screening in pregnancy and perinatal morbidity in infants of mothers with mild impairment in glucose tolerance. *Diabetes Care*. 1980;3:447–452.
4. Beischer NA, Oats JN, Henry OA, Sheedy MT, Walstab JE. Incidence and severity of gestational diabetes mellitus according to country of birth in women living in Australia. *Diabetes*. 1991;40(Suppl. 2):S35-S38.
5. National Diabetes Data Group. Classification and diagnosis of diabetes mellitus and other categories of glucose intolerance. *Diabetes*. 1979;28:1039–1057.
6. World Health Organization. *Diabetes Mellitus: Report of a WHO Study Group*. Geneva, Switzerland: World Health Organization; 1985. Technical Report Series 727.
7. Malecki MT, Moczulski DK, Klupa T, Wanic K, Cyganek K, Frey J, Sieradzki J. Homozygous combination of calpain 10 gene haplotypes is associated with type 2 diabetes mellitus in a Polish population. *Eur J Endocrinol*. 2002;146:695–699.
8. Gower BA, Fernandez JR, Beasley TM, Shrive MD, Goran MI. Using genetic admixture to explain racial differences in insulin-related phenotypes. *Diabetes*. 2003;52:1047–1051.

9. Williams RC, Long JC, Hanson RL, Sievers ML, Knowler WC. Individual estimates of European genetic admixture associated with lower body mass index, plasma glucose, and prevalence of type 2 diabetes in Pima Indians. *Am J Hum Genet.* 2000;66:527–538.

10. Reitmauer PJ, Go RC, Acton RT, Murphy CC, Budowle B, Barger BO, Roseman JM. Evidence for genetic admixture as a determinant in the occurrence of insulin-dependent diabetes mellitus in U.S. blacks. *Diabetes.* 1982;31:532–537.

11. Mitchell BD, Valdez R, Hazuda HP, Haffner SM, Monterrosa A, Stern MP. Differences in the prevalence of diabetes and impaired glucose tolerance according to maternal or paternal history of diabetes. *Diabetes Care.* 1993;16:1262–1267.

12. Gutierrez YM. Cultural factors affecting diet and pregnancy outcome of Mexican American adolescents. *J Adolesc Health.* 1999;25:227–237.

13. Gutierrez YM. *Cultural Factors Affecting Diet and Pregnancy Outcome of Mexican American Adolescents* [PhD dissertation]. Berkeley, Calif: Department of Nutritional Science/Natural Resources, University of California, Berkeley; 1995.

14. McNeely MJ, Boyko EJ, Shofer JB, Newell-Morris L, Leonetti DL, Fugimoto WY. Standard definitions of overweight and central adiposity for determining diabetes risk in Japanese Americans. *Am J Clin Nutr.* 2001;74:101–107.

15. Marshall JA, Hamman RF, Baxter J, Mayer EJ, Fulton DL, Orleans M, Rewers M, Jones RH. Ethnic differences in risk factors associated with the prevalence of non-insulin dependent diabetes mellitus. The San Luis Valley Diabetes Study. *Am J Epidemiol.* 1993;137:706–718.

16. Schorlin JB, Saunders JT. Is "sugar" the same as diabetes? A community based study among rural African-Americans. *Diabetes Care.* 2000;23:330–334.

17. Health Resources and Services Administration Bureau of Health Professions Division of Nursing. Other definitions of cultural competence. Available at: http://bhpr.hrsa.gov/diversity/cultcomp.htm. Accessed December 7, 2004.

18. Health Resources and Services Administration. Cultural competence works: using cultural competence to improve the quality of health care for diverse populations and add value to managed care arrangements. Available at: http://www.hrsa.gov/financeMC/ftp/cultural-competence.pdf. Accessed December 7, 2004.

19. Berlin EA, Fowkes WC Jr. A teaching framework for cross-cultural health care. Application in family practice. *West J Med.* 1983;139:934–938.

20. Like RC, Steiner RP, Rubel AJ. STFM core curriculum guidelines. recommended core curriculum guidelines on culturally sensitive and competent health care. *Fam Med.* 1996;28:291–297.

21. American Dietetic Association. NCND bibliography on ethnic food habits. Available at: http://www.eatright.org/public/other/index_biibethnic.cfm. Accessed December 7, 2004.

22. *Dietary Guidelines for Americans 2005.* Available at: http://www.healthierus.gov/dietaryguidelines. Accessed May 3, 2005.

23. Melville MB, ed. *Twice a Minority: Mexican-American Women.* St. Louis, Mo: Mosby; 1980.

10

Postpartum Considerations

Yolanda M. Gutierrez, MS, PhD, RD, and Alyce M. Thomas, RD

OBJECTIVES   After completing this chapter, you will be able to do the following:

1. Discuss postpartum screening and diagnosis procedures for women with gestational diabetes mellitus (GDM).
2. Present the uses of medical nutrition therapy and other risk-reducing strategies for women with a history of GDM.
3. Explain the benefits of breastfeeding for women with gestational diabetes mellitus (GDM).
4. Discuss the nutrition requirements of postpartum women with previous GDM.
5. Describe the long-term health risks associated with GDM.

POSTPARTUM SCREENING AND DIAGNOSIS

The American Diabetes Association recommends postpartum screening (usually performed 6 weeks after delivery) for all women with previous GDM (1). The purpose of postpartum screening is to identify women who are likely to have diabetes (2).

In women with a history of GDM, reassessment of glycemic levels should be repeated every 3 years (1). Women with impaired fasting glucose or impaired glucose tolerance should be tested annually. The American Diabetes Association recommends fasting plasma glucose as the best screening test for diabetes because of its ease and convenience (3). ACOG suggests that if the results of the oral glucose tolerance test (OGTT) and fasting plasma glucose are normal, then fasting plasma glucose may be used as the follow-up test (4). Jacob Reichelt et al found that, although the fasting plasma glucose identified approximately 90% of women with diabetes, only 25% would have been detected using the im-

TABLE 10.1 Criteria for Diagnosis of Diabetes Mellitus After Pregnancy

	Normal Values, mg/dL (mmol/L)	Impaired Fasting Glucose, mg/dL (mmol/L)	Impaired Glucose Tolerance, mg/dL (mmol/L)	Diabetes Mellitus, mg/dL (mmol/L)
Fasting plasma glucose	<100 (<5.6)	≥100 to <126 (≥5.6 to <7.8)	<100 (<5.6)	≥126 (≥7.0)
75-g OGTT	<140 (7.8)	<140 (7.8)	≥140 to <200 (≥7.8 to <11.1)	≥200 (11.8)

Abbreviation: OGTT, oral glucose tolerance test.
Source: Adapted with permission from American Diabetes Association. Screening for type 2 diabetes. *Diabetes Care.* 2004;27(Suppl 1):S11–S14.

paired glucose tolerance criteria (5). If the results of the OGTT are abnormal, it is possible that the woman had undiagnosed diabetes before conception (see Chapter 3).

As outlined in Table 10.1, the criteria for diagnosing diabetes after pregnancy are based on the American Diabetes Association's position statement on screening for type 2 diabetes (3). If the results of the tests indicate type 2 diabetes, the woman is to be referred for diabetes education, including medical nutrition therapy (MNT) (see Chapter 6).

PREVENTION OF TYPE 2 DIABETES IN WOMEN WITH GESTATIONAL DIABETES

Women with a history of GDM are at increased risk of developing diabetes (usually type 2) in the future (6,7). Research suggests that calculations of the risk of future type 2 diabetes depend on the diagnostic criteria used to identify GDM and maternal risk factors (8). Certain risk factors for type 2 diabetes may be modifiable in women with GDM during the postpartum period. These risk factors include obesity, future weight gain, level of physical activity, and breastfeeding. There are, however, risk factors that cannot be modified postpartum, including ethnicity, pre-pregnancy weight, age, parity, family history of diabetes, and degree of hyperglycemia in pregnancy and immediately after delivery (6,7,9–11).

There is evidence to suggest that some women with a history of GDM show relative β-cell dysfunction during and after pregnancy (12,13). Most women with a history of GDM are insulin resistant (14,15). To this extent, changes in lifestyle may improve postpartum insulin sensitivity and could possibly preserve β-cell function to slow the progression of type 2 diabetes (14). The Diabetes Prevention Program Research Group concluded that type 2 diabetes can be prevented or delayed in persons at high risk for the disease, such as women with a history of GDM, by making lifestyle changes (16). In this study, 3,234 persons with diabetes were randomized into three groups: lifestyle modification, metformin, and placebo. Those in the lifestyle intervention group received individual counseling, which included a goal to achieve or maintain a weight reduction of at least 7% of their initial body weight, low-calorie, low-fat diet instruction, and the adoption of moderate physical activity for at least 150 minutes per week. The lifestyle intervention group reduced their incidence of type 2 diabetes by 58%, compared with a reduction of 31% in the metformin group (16).

Body Weight and Obesity

There is strong evidence that obesity, weight gain, and physical inactivity are the main modifiable risk factors in the development of type 2 diabetes (17). Women who lose weight to reach and maintain their ideal body weight significantly decrease their risk of developing type 2 diabetes; and studies suggest that type 2 diabetes can be delayed or prevented with only modest weight loss (17,18). In the Finnish Diabetes Prevention study (17), women in the intervention group received individualized counseling, which emphasized weight reduction, a decrease in total fat and saturated fat intake, and an increase in fiber intake. They averaged more weight loss (4.2 ± 5.1 kg) than women in the control group (0.8 ± 3.7 kg), which received only general oral and written information on diet and exercise (17). Long et al (19) reported that obese subjects with impaired glucose tolerance delayed their progression to type 2 diabetes by losing weight.

The increase of visceral fat in obese individuals may be one reason why obesity can trigger type 2 diabetes. Central obesity, as estimated indirectly by skin folds or waist-to-hip ratio, is a predictive factor for type 2 diabetes (20). Insulin sensitivity improves with weight loss, increasing to a greater extent when abdominal fat and waist-to-hip ratio decreases (21).

Dietetics professionals can play an important role in helping women manage weight after delivery. According to the American Dietetic Association's 2002 position statement on weight management, an assessment of the woman's weight and health status is necessary to determine the goals of treatment (22). The assessment consists of the following parameters:

- *Anthropometric:* Measuring height, current weight, body mass index (BMI), and waist circumference
- *Medical:* Identifying potential causes, associated disorders, and severity of obesity
- *Psychological:* Assessing the barriers to treatment
- *Nutritional:* Determining weight history, diet history, current eating pattern, nutrition intake, environmental factors, exercise history, and the woman's motivation for and readiness to change

Physical Activity

Exercise has a beneficial effect on insulin action by enhancing peripheral tissue glucose uptake (23). Additional improvement in insulin action may be realized by decreasing body weight through regular exercise and diet and by ameliorating the detrimental effect of inactivity on insulin sensitivity (24).

Mild to vigorous exercise performed regularly has the potential to reduce the risk of type 2 diabetes by 30% to 50% (25). Manson et al observed a reduced incidence of type 2 diabetes among women who exercised regularly when compared with their sedentary counterparts (26). Fulton-Kehoe et al studied the impact of physical activity on Hispanic and non-Hispanic subjects (27). The results suggested that persons with higher levels of physical activity were 25% to 50% less likely to develop type 2 diabetes.

The benefits of exercise extend to both obese and nonobese women. When counseling women about physical activity, dietetics professionals should recommend at least 30 minutes per day of moderate physical activity, for maximum effects. If the woman is unable to exercise at a moderate pace, a higher activity level for a shorter period of time can be just as effective.

MEDICAL NUTRITION THERAPY

MNT is an essential component in the care of women with previous GDM. Nutrition intervention may delay or prevent the onset of diabetes later in life (1,28).

The goals of MNT for women with previous GDM are based on recommendations from the American Diabetes Association (28). The recommendations, similar to those for MNT for type 2 diabetes, are designed to decrease the risk of developing type 2 diabetes.

Carbohydrate and monounsaturated fat intake should comprise 60% of the total daily calories, with the remainder as protein. It may be necessary to adjust energy intake to achieve an ideal body weight. Saturated fat intake should be less than 10% of the total energy, and dietary cholesterol should be less than 300 mg/day. The consumption of whole grains, fruits, and vegetables is encouraged, to increase the fiber intake and to promote glycemic control. A modification of the individualized pregnancy meal plan may be an ideal plan for women with a history of GDM (28).

When counseling women about dietary choices after delivery, emphasis should be placed on limiting fat intake and choosing heart-healthy fats. Studies have shown that a diet higher in fat, especially from animal sources, is associated with an earlier diagnosis of type 2 diabetes in comparison with lower-fat diets (14,29). The type of fat consumed is also a factor in the risk of developing type 2 diabetes; saturated fat intake is thought to increase risk the most (28). Moses reported that the recurrence of GDM was greater when women consumed more fat between pregnancies (30). The prevalence of type 2 diabetes increased when the energy from fat intake exceeded 40% of total energy (31). Population studies show that high-fat diets are often associated with hyperinsulinemia, which suggests that an increased and long-standing insulin resistance would have an adverse cumulative effect on β-cell reserve, increasing the risk for type 2 diabetes (31–33).

BREASTFEEDING

Breastfeeding has been shown to lower the blood glucose level and to decrease the incidence of type 2 diabetes in women with a history of GDM (34–36). It is also associated with weight loss and reduced insulin resistance (37,38).

Weight-Loss Benefits

Breastfeeding can assist women in losing weight if they do not increase energy intake during the postpartum period. The estimated milk energy output is approximately 500 kcal/day in the first 6 months and 400 kcal/day in the second 6 months of lactation (39). The estimated energy requirements (EERs) for lactation are as follows (39):

- Age 14–18 years: EER = Adolescent EER + Milk Energy Output – Weight Loss
  First 6 months = Adolescent EER + 500 – 170 (Milk Energy Output – Weight Loss)
  Second 6 months = Adolescent EER + 400 – 0 (Milk Energy Output – Weight Loss)

- Age 19–50 years: EER = Adult EER + Milk Energy Output – Weight Loss
  First 6 months = Adult EER + 500 – 170 (Milk Energy Output – Weight Loss)
  Second 6 months = Adult EER + 400 – 0 (Milk Energy Output – Weight Loss)

Beneficial Effects on Glucose Metabolism

The need for glucose in the synthesis of breastmilk is one possible reason for which breastfeeding may lower maternal blood glucose levels. Lactose is the only carbohydrate found in breastmilk, and it requires glucose for synthesis and the volume of milk produced. The estimated mean concentration of lactose in mature breastmilk is 72 g/L (40). Lactose is composed of one molecule of glucose and one molecule of galactose. Because galactose is synthesized from glucose, both monosaccharides in lactose are essentially derived from glucose (41). Glucose in the mammary gland is derived primarily from plasma glucose. Lactose synthesis increases glucose utilization by 30% in exclusively breastfeeding women (42). Additionally, glucose is needed as a source of fuel for energy utilization in lactating women (43–45).

Few studies have addressed the effects of breastfeeding on blood glucose concentrations in women with type 1 diabetes (46–50), and even fewer have focused on breastfeeding and women with previous GDM (36,50). Kjos et al reported on the effects of lactation on glucose metabolism in 809 women with recent GDM (36). Approximately half of the women (404) breastfed their infants; the other 405 women did not breastfeed. Using a 2-hour, 75-g OGTT performed at 4 to 12 weeks after delivery, the authors found that breastfeeding women had improved glucose tolerance, as indicated by a significantly lower area under the glucose curve, with fasting and 2-hour glucose levels lower than the nonlactating group. The study, however, did not include the number of women who breastfed for 4 weeks or for 12 weeks.

A study by Yang et al (50) comparing the regular insulin requirements of breastfeeding and non-breastfeeding Chinese women with type 1 diabetes or GDM found that regular insulin requirements decreased significantly in the postpartum period when the women with type 1 diabetes breastfed their infants. Of the 10 women with GDM who breastfed, 7 did not require regular insulin during the postpartum period. Three women with GDM who did not breastfeed required regular insulin for 4 to 7 days after delivery.

Nutrition Recommendations

Daily Nutrient Requirements

The nutrition needs of lactating women who had GDM in pregnancy are the same as for lactating women who do not have diabetes. Daily nutrient requirements are outlined in Table 10.2 (39,51–54).

Nutrition-Related Factors and the Composition of Breastmilk

Several nutrition-related factors can alter the composition of breastmilk (55). For example, a woman's prenatal nutrition, the amount of weight gained during pregnancy, nutrient intake, and changes in her eating habits (eg, seasonal shifts, disease-related adaptations, supplements, dieting) all can affect human milk composition.

Key points to understand about the relationship between the diet of the lactating woman and the composition of breastmilk include the following recommendations from the Institute of Medicine (55):

- Increases in saturated and unsaturated fatty acids in the diet increase the concentration of these nutrients in breast milk.
- Diet does not seem to alter the concentration of cholesterol and phospholipids in human milk.
- A diet consisting of fewer than 1,500 kcal/day has been shown to decrease milk volume in lactating women.
- The content of certain nutrients in human milk may be maintained at a satisfactory level at the expense of maternal stores. This applies particularly to folate and calcium.
- As a general rule, vitamin concentration in breastmilk is dependent on intake/maternal stores. Concentrations of major minerals (calcium, phosphorus, magnesium, sodium, potassium) in human milk may not be affected by diet. The effects of diet on concentrations of other minerals (selenium, iron, zinc) are unknown.

TABLE 10.2 Daily Nutrient Requirements During Lactation

Nutrient (References)	Nonpregnant Women, Age 15–50 y	Lactation
Energy, kcal (39)	2200	+500
Protein, g (39)	46	+25
Vitamin A, µg RAE (51)	700	Age 14–18 y: 1200
		Age 19–50 y: 770
Vitamin D, µg (52)	5	5
Vitamin K, µg (51)	90	Age 14–18 y: 75
		Age 19–50 y: 90
Vitamin C, mg (53)	75	Age 14–18 y: 115
		Age 19–50 y: 120
Thiamin, mg (54)	1.1	1.4
Riboflavin, mg (54)	1.1	1.6
Niacin, mg NE (54)	14	17
Vitamin B-6, mg (54)	1.3	2.0
Folate, µg FE (54)	400	500
Vitamin B-12, µg (54)	2.4	2.8
Calcium, mg (52)	1000	Age 14–18 y: 1300
		Age 19–50 y: 1000
Phosphorus, mg (52)	700	Age 14–18 y: 1250
		Age 19–50 y: 700
Magnesium, mg (52)	360–265	Age 14–18 y: 360
		Age 19–50 y: 320
Iron, mg (51)	18	Age 14–18 y: 10
		Age 19–50 y: 9
Zinc, mg (51)	8	Age 14–18 y: 13
		Age 19–50 y: 12
Iodine, µg (51)	150	290
Selenium, µg (53)	55	70

Obstacles to Breastfeeding

Dietetics professionals and other practitioners should be prepared to help women address a variety of possible challenges to successful breastfeeding. For example, the initiation of lactation may be delayed by a cesarean section. Being separated from the baby, infrequent feedings, and supplemental feedings are other factors that may make it difficult to initiate or continue breastfeeding.

Women diagnosed with type 2 diabetes after having GDM require special education concerning breastfeeding, especially with regard to maintaining blood glucose control. The education should include the use of oral hypoglycemic agents, nutrition needs, blood glucose control, and family planning. For nutrition recommendations for breastfeeding, see Box 10.1.

LONG-TERM HEALTH RISKS

The birth of the infant brings an end to many, but not all, of the complications associated with GDM. A history of GDM is a risk factor for developing type 2 diabetes and for devel-

BOX 10.1

Nutrition Advice for Breastfeeding After Gestational Diabetes Mellitus

- Eat three meals and three or more snacks per day.
- Choose a variety of foods every day.
- Include three or more daily servings from the milk group.
- Drink to satisfy thirst only. Excess fluids have no benefit on breastmilk production.
- Strive for slow weight loss on an individualized meal plan designed by the dietetics professional.
- Use daily multivitamins with iron. Supplements do not replace all the nutrients needed by lactating women.
- Limit coffee, tea, and other caffeine-containing beverages to 1 cup per day.
- Keep extra portions of food in the freezer for future use, and do not ignore offers from family and friends to help with meals.
- Use nonnutritive sweeteners in moderation (<4 servings/day).

oping GDM in subsequent pregnancies. If a woman's lipid levels are elevated, a history of GDM is also a risk factor for cardiovascular disorders.

Risk for Type 2 Diabetes

In approximately 60% of women with previous GDM, type 2 diabetes will be diagnosed during the 5 to 15 years after the pregnancy, depending on the racial or ethnic group. Factors associated with impaired glucose tolerance and type 2 diabetes in women with a history of GDM include age of the mother, obesity, abnormally high glycemic levels during the OGTT in pregnancy and postpartum, and diagnosis of GDM before 24 weeks' gestation (4). Women with GDM should be informed of the potential risks for the progression of GDM to type 2 diabetes and the long-term risks of developing type 2 diabetes (35,56–59). The importance of primary preventive health care for all women, with or without diabetes, must be a priority for all health care providers.

Risk of Recurrence of GDM in Subsequent Pregnancies

The risk of developing GDM in a subsequent pregnancy in women with previous GDM is 30% to 65% (14,28,60,61). Preterm delivery and elevated fasting glycemic levels are predictors for the development of diabetes in women with previous GDM (58). In a study to determine the incidence of the development of diabetes with a previous history of GDM, Damm et al (58) compared glucose tolerance in 241 women with previous GDM (diet controlled) with a control group of 57 women with normoglycemia during pregnancy. While no one in the control group developed diabetes, 42 of the women with previous GDM developed diabetes (3.7% with type 1 diabetes and 13.7% with type 2 diabetes.

Factors that increase the risk of recurrent GDM include the amount of weight gained between pregnancies, hip-to-waist ratio, and diet composition (5,62). In a study by Lu et al (63) to determine the incidence of GDM in a subsequent pregnancy in women who did not develop GDM in their first pregnancy, women who were obese (BMI > 29.2), had a 1-hour glucose challenge test of more than 101 mg/dL and those who gained more than 5 kg between pregnancies were more likely to develop GDM in subsequent pregnancies (odds ratio, 2.2; 95% CI, 1.1–4.5) than women who gained less than 4.7 kg between pregnancies. None of the women who gained less than 4.7 kg developed GDM in subsequent pregnancies. A Brazilian study (5) found that women who were short in stature (<154 cm) and had high hip-to-waist ratios (>0.84) when diagnosed with GDM were at greater risk for developing future glucose abnormalities. The researchers concluded that women with previous GDM had twice the risk of developing diabetes or impaired glucose intolerance 4 to 8 years after pregnancy than control subjects without GDM (5). Moses et al (62) compared the dietary fat intake of women with recurring GDM to that of a control group without GDM recurrence. Women with recurring GDM consumed almost 40% of their energy from fat compared with 34% in the control group.

Cardiovascular Disease Risk

Pallardo et al (64) examined the association of cardiovascular risk factors and impaired fasting glucose and impaired glucose tolerance in women with a history of GDM. Higher incidences of increased diastolic blood pressure and triglycerides were found in women with impaired fasting glucose and impaired glucose tolerance values than in women with normal glycemic levels. The researchers concluded that impaired glucose metabolism was significantly associated with cardiovascular risk factors.

ADDITIONAL CONSIDERATIONS

Preconception Counseling

More than 50% of pregnancies in the United States are unplanned, and this statistic suggests that all women with a history of GDM can benefit greatly from preconception counseling (63). If a woman was diagnosed in a previous pregnancy with GDM, a 75-g OGTT should be performed to screen for diabetes or impaired glucose tolerance before conception; if preconception screening was not performed, the woman should be screened at the first prenatal visit (3). If type 2 diabetes has developed since the last pregnancy, counseling should focus on the risks of abnormal maternal glycemic levels to the fetus, especially in early pregnancy. Every effort must be undertaken to achieve normal blood glucose levels, beginning 3 months before conception through the critical first 10 weeks after conception.

Obese women should be encouraged to lose weight before conception (14). Sufficient calcium intake may help in weight loss. Zemel et al (65) found that obese adults following a reduced-energy diet high in calcium (1,200–1,300 mg/day) lost more weight and fat than those on a reduced-energy, low-calcium (400–500 mg/day) diet. The impact of calcium on weight loss is even greater when the mineral is supplied by low-fat dairy products rather than from calcium supplements. Researchers have not yet determined the reason(s) for the enhanced effect of dairy products, although it is known that other nutrients present in foods, such as proteins, vitamin D, and magnesium, enhance calcium absorption (65).

Women should be advised that additional lifestyle changes that could affect fetal development and outcome, such as stopping the use of alcohol, tobacco, and other harmful substances, need to be instituted before conception is attempted (66). (See Chapter 8.) Multivitamin-mineral supplementation should be assessed to avoid possible teratogenic effects on fetal development. A supplement containing more than the Tolerable Upper Limit for vitamins and minerals is not recommended (see Chapter 7).

Contraception

The issue of family planning is important in the care of women with a history of GDM. A discussion of family planning should be part of the postpartum visit to the health care provider, along with a complete physical and gynecological examination.

Contraceptive methods include barrier methods, intrauterine (IUDs), or oral contraceptives. No adverse effects have been associated with the barrier method used by women with diabetes. IUDs are not usually prescribed for women with diabetes, because of the higher risk of adverse effects, including heavier menses and infection (67). Oral contraceptive use in women with a history of GDM is controversial. Adverse effects (thromboembolism, myocardial infarction, stroke) associated with oral contraceptives could increase the risk of cardiovascular disease in these women (67–69). There is an increased risk of insulin resistance associated with oral contraceptive use, which may be caused by a reduction in the concentration of insulin receptors (67). Progesterone-only oral contraceptives are not recommended for women with a history of GDM, because of increased insulin resistance and its effect on high-density lipoprotein levels (67). Kjos et al showed that progesterone-only oral contraceptives significantly increased the risk of developing type 2 diabetes in women with an abnormal OGTT during pregnancy (68). The lowest dose of estrogen and progesterone should be prescribed for women with diabetes (69).

Very little information is available on the use of long-acting progestins in women with a history of GDM. Norplant (Wyeth Laboratories, Philadelphia, PA 19101), a progesterone-based contraceptive, releases levonorgestrel into the bloodstream and is associated with increased glucose and insulin levels in women without diabetes (69). Medroxyprogesterone acetate (Depo-Provera [Pharmacia & Upjohn Company, Kalamazoo, MI 49001]) was reported to limit carbohydrate tolerance and should not be used in women with a history of GDM (70). Depo-Provera is also associated with decreased levels of serum triglycerides and high-density lipoproteins (70). If a woman decides to use the long-acting progestins, periodic glucose and lipid assessments are necessary.

SUMMARY

Postpartum screening and diagnosis of women with GDM can help identify women at greater risk of developing diabetes or other health problems. There are strategies to help prevent the development of diabetes. Women with diabetes during pregnancy should be encouraged to breastfeed their infants. Studies indicate that breastfeeding may have a beneficial effect on postpartum glycemic levels in women with previous GDM. Most women with a history of GDM are insulin resistant, both during and after pregnancy. Lifestyle changes may improve insulin sensitivity during the postpartum period, which may slow the progression of type 2 diabetes (16). In 2002, the Diabetes Prevention Program Research Group concluded that type 2 diabetes can be prevented or delayed in persons at high risk for the disease, such as women with a history of GDM, by making lifestyle changes. Obesity, future weight gain, level of physical activity, and breastfeeding are risk factors that can be modified. Results from research suggest that lifestyle changes may reduce the incidence of diabetes by 58% (17).

The nutrition needs of lactating women with previous GDM are similar to those of lactating women without diabetes. There are issues that may challenge the success of breastfeeding. Research continues to explore how breastfeeding protects women from diabetes. Health care providers have the responsibility to encourage, promote, educate, and support women and their families for a successful lactation experience.

Women should discuss contraceptive methods with their health care providers. Preconception counseling is highly recommended for women with a history of GDM, to improve future pregnancy outcomes.

REFERENCES

1. American Diabetes Association. Gestational diabetes mellitus. *Diabetes Care.* 2004;27(Suppl 1):S88–S90.

2. Sherwin RS, Anderson RM, Buse JB, Chin MH, Eddy D, Fradkin J, Ganiats TG, Ginsberg H, Kahn R, Nwankwo R, Rewers M, Schlessinger L, Stern M, Vinicor F, Zinman B; American Diabetes Association. The prevention or delay of type 2 diabetes. *Diabetes Care.* 2003;26(Suppl 1):S62–S69.

3. American Diabetes Association. Screening for type 2 diabetes. *Diabetes Care.* 2004;27(Suppl 1):S11–S14.

4. American College of Obstetricians and Gynecologists Committee on Practice Bulletins—Obstetrics. ACOG Practice Bulletin. Clinical management guidelines for obstetrician-gynecologists. Number 30, September 2001 (replaces Technical Bulletin Number 200, December 1994). Gestational diabetes. *Obstet Gynecol.* 2001;98:525–538.

5. Jacob Reichelt AA, Ferraz TM, Rocha Oppermann ML, Costa e Forti A, Duncan BB, Fleck Pessoa E, Schmidt MI. Detecting glucose intolerance after gestational diabetes: inadequacy of fasting glucose alone and risk associated with gestational diabetes and second trimester waist-hip ratio. *Diabetologia.* 2002;45:455–457.

6. Metzger BE, Cho NH, Roston SM, Radvany R. Prepregnancy weight and antepartum insulin secretion predict glucose tolerance five years after gestational diabetes mellitus. *Diabetes Care.* 1993;16:1598–1605.

7. Kjos SL, Peters RK, Xiang A, Henry OA, Montoro M, Buchanan TA. Predicting future diabetes in Latino women with gestational diabetes. Utility of early postpartum glucose tolerance testing. *Diabetes.* 1995;44:586–591.

8. Metzger BE, Bybee DE, Freinkel N, Phelps RL, Radvany RM, Vaisrub N. Gestational diabetes mellitus: correlations between the phenotypic and genotypic characteristics of the mother and abnormal glucose tolerance during the first year postpartum. *Diabetes.* 1985;34(Suppl 2):S111–S115.

9. Berkowitz GS, Lapinski RH, Wein R, Lee D. Race/ethnicity and other risk factors for gestational diabetes. *Am J Epidemiol.* 1992;135:965–973.

10. Dornhorst A, Paterson CM, Nicholls JS, Wadsworth J, Chiu DC, Elkeles RS, Johnston DG, Beard RW. High prevalence of gestational diabetes in women from ethnic minority groups. *Diabete Med.* 1992;9:820–825.

11. Henry OA, Beischer NA. Long-term complications of gestational diabetes for the mother. *Baillieres Clin Obstet Gynecol.* 1991;5:461–483.

12. Buchanan TA, Metzger BE, Frienkel N, Bergman RN. Insulin sensitivity and β-cell responsiveness to glucose during late pregnancy in lean and moderately obese women with normal glucose tolerance and mild gestational diabetes. *Am J Obstet Gynecol.* 1990; 162:1008–1014.

13. Dornhorst A, Bailey PC, Anyaoku V, Elkeles RS, Johnston DG, Beard RW. Abnormalities of glucose tolerance following gestational diabetes. *Q J Med.* 1990;77:1219–1228.

14. Dornhorst A, Frost G. The potential for dietary intervention postpartum in women with gestational diabetes. *Diabetes Care.* 1997;20:1635–1637.

15. Ryan EA, Imes S, Liu D, McManus R, Finegood DT, Polonsky KS, Sturis J. Defects in insulin secretion and action in women with a history of gestational diabetes. *Diabetes.* 1995;44:506–512.

16. Knowler WC, Barrett-Connor E, Fowler SE, Hamman RF, Lachin JM, Walker EA, Nathan DM; Diabetes Prevention Program Research Group. Reduction in the incidence of type 2 diabetes with lifestyle intervention or metformin. *N Engl J Med.* 2002;346:393–403.

17. Tuomilehto J, Lindstrom J, Eriksson JG, Valle TT, Hamalainen H, Ilanne-Parikka P, Keinanen-Kiukaanniemi S, Laakso M, Louheranta A, Rastas M, Salminen V, Uusitupa M; Finnish Diabetes

Prevention Study Group. Prevention of type 2 diabetes mellitus by changes in lifestyle among subjects with impaired glucose tolerance. *N Engl J Med.* 2001;344:1343–1350.

18. Dornhorst A, Rossi M. Risks and prevention of type 2 diabetes in women with gestational diabetes. *Diabetes Care.* 1998;21(Suppl 2):B43–B49.

19. Long SD, O'Brien K, MacDonald KG Jr, Leggett-Frazier N, Swanson MS, Pories WJ, Caro JF. Weight loss in severely obese subjects prevents the progression of impaired glucose tolerance to type 2 diabetes. A longitudinal interventional study. *Diabetes Care.* 1994;17:372–375.

20. Ohlson LO, Larsson B, Svardsudd K, Welin L, Eriksson H, Wilhelmsen L, Bjorntorp P, Tibblin G. The influence of body fat distribution on the incidence of diabetes mellitus. *Diabetes.* 1985;34:1055–1058.

21. Holte J, Bergh T, Berne C, Wide L, Lithell H. Restored insulin sensitivity but persistently increased early insulin secretion after weight loss in obese women with polycystic ovary syndrome. *J Clin Endocrinol Metab.* 1995;80:2586–2593.

22. Cummings S, Parham ES, Strain GW; American Dietetic Association. Position of the American Dietetic Association: weight management. *J Am Diet Assoc.* 2002;102:1145–1155.

23. Hollenbeck CB, Haskell W, Rosenthal M, Reaven GM. Effect of habitual physical activity on regulation of insulin-stimulated glucose disposal in older males. *J Am Geriatr Soc.* 1985;33:273–277.

24. Eriksson J, Taimela S, Koivisto VA. Exercise and the metabolic syndrome. *Diabetologia.* 1997;40:125–135.

25. Manson JE, Spelsberg A. Primary prevention of non-insulin-dependent diabetes mellitus. *Am J Prev Med.* 1994;10:172–184.

26. Manson JE, Rimm EB, Stampfer MJ, Colditz GA, Willett WC, Krolewski AS, Rosner B, Hennekens CH, Speizer FE. Physical activity and incidence of non-insulin-dependent diabetes mellitus in women. *Lancet.* 1991;338:774–778.

27. Fulton-Kehoe D, Hamman RF, Baxter J, Marshall J. A case-control study of physical activity and non-insulin dependent diabetes mellitus (NIDDM). The San Luis Valley Diabetes Study. *Ann Epidemiol.* 2001;11:320–327.

28. Franz MJ, Bantle JP, Beebe CA, Brunzell JD, Chiasson JL, Garg A, Holzmeister LA, Hoogwerf B, Mayer-Davis E, Mooradian AD, Purnell JQ, Wheeler M; American Diabetes Association. Evidence-based nutrition principles and recommendations for the treatment and prevention of diabetes and related complications. *Diabetes Care.* 2003;26(Suppl 1):S51–S61.

29. Mayer-Davis EJ, Monaco JH, Hoen HM, Carmichael S, Vitolins MZ, Rewers MJ, Haffner SM, Ayad MF, Bergman RN, Karter AJ. Dietary fat and insulin sensitivity in a triethnic population: the role of obesity. The Insulin Resistance Atherosclerosis Study (IRAS). *Am J Clin Nutr.* 1997;65:79–87.

30. Moses RG. The recurrence rate of gestational diabetes in subsequent pregnancies. *Diabetes Care.* 1996;19:1348–1350.

31. Marshall JA, Hamman RF, Baxter J. High-fat, low-carbohydrate diet and the etiology of non-insulin-dependent diabetes mellitus: the San Luis Valley Diabetes Study. *Am J Epidemiol.* 1991;134:590–603.

32. Marshall JA, Bessesen DH, Hamman RF. High saturated fat and low starch and fibre are associated with hyperinsulinaemia in a non-diabetic population: the San Luis Valley Diabetes Study. *Diabetologia.* 1997;40:430–438.

33. Feskens EJ, Virtanen SM, Rasanen L, Tuomilehto J, Stengard J, Pekkanen J, Nissinen A, Kromhout D. Dietary factors determining diabetes and impaired glucose tolerance. A 20-year follow-up of the Finnish and Dutch cohorts of the Seven Countries Study. *Diabetes Care.* 1995;18:1104–1112.

34. Kjos SL, Buchanan TA. Gestational diabetes mellitus. *New Engl J Med.* 1999;341:1749–1756.

35. Kjos SL. Postpartum care of the woman with diabetes. *Clin Obstet Gynecol.* 2000;43:75–86.

36. Kjos SL, Henry O, Lee RM, Buchanan TA, Mishell DR Jr. The effect of lactation on glucose and lipid metabolism in women with recent gestational diabetes. *Obstet Gynecol.* 1993;82:451–455.

37. Brewer MM, Bates MR, Vannoy LP. Postpartum changes in maternal weight and body fat depots in lactating vs nonlactating women. *Am J Clin Nutr.* 1989;49:259–265.

38. Dewey KG, Heinig MJ, Nommsen LA. Maternal weight-loss patterns during prolonged lactation. *Am J Clin Nutr.* 1993;58:162–166.

39. Institute of Medicine. *Dietary Reference Intakes for Energy, Carbohydrate, Fiber, Fat, Fatty Acids, Cholesterol, Protein, and Amino Acids (Macronutrients).* Washington, DC: National Academy Press; 2002.

40. McGanity WJ, Dawson EB, Van Hook JW. Maternal nutrition. In: Shils ME, Olson JA, Shine M Ross AC. eds. *Modern Nutrition in Health and Disease.* Baltimore, Md: Williams and Wilkins; 1998:811–838.

41. Nelson DL, Lehninger AL, Cox MM. *Principles of Biochemistry.* 2nd ed. New York, NY: Worth Publishers; 1993.

42. Lawrence RA, Lawrence RM. *Breastfeeding: A Guide for the Medical Profession.* 5th ed. St. Louis, Mo: Mosby; 1999.

43. Food and Agriculture Organization, World Health Organization, and United Nations University. Energy and protein requirements. Report of a joint FAO/WHO/UNU Expert Consultation. *World Health Organ Tech Rep Ser.* 1985;724:1–206.

44. van Raaij JM, Schonk CM, Vermaat-Miedema SH, Peek ME, Hautvast JG. Energy cost of lactation, and energy balances of well-nourished Dutch lactating women: reappraisal of the extra energy requirements of lactation. *Am J Clin Nutr.* 1991;53:612–619.

45. Butte NF, Wong WW, Hopkinson JM. Energy requirements of lactating women derived from doubly labeled water and milk energy output. *J Nutr.* 2001;131:53–58.

46. Davies HA, Clark JD, Dalton KJ, Edwards OM. Insulin requirements of diabetic women who breast feed. *BMJ.* 1989;298:1357–1358.

47. Whichelow MJ, Doddridge MC. Lactation in diabetic women. *Br Med J (Clin Res Ed).* 1983;287:649–650.

48. Ferris AM, Dalidowitz CK, Ingardia CM, Reece EA, Fumia FD, Jensen RG, Allen LA. Lactation outcome in insulin-dependent diabetic women. *J Am Diet Assoc.* 1988;88:317–322.

49. Murtaugh MA, Ferris AM, Capacchione CM, Reece EA. Energy intake and glycemia in lactation women with type 1 diabetes. *J Am Diet Assoc.* 1998;98:642–648.

50. Yang JQ, Xu YH, Gai MY. Breastfeeding in reducing regular insulin requirements in postpartum for insulin dependent diabetes mellitus and gestational diabetes. *Zhoghua Fu Chan Ke Za Zhi.* 1994;29:135, 137, 138.

51. Institute of Medicine. *Dietary Reference Intakes for Vitamin A, Vitamin K, Arsenic, Boron, Chromium, Copper, Iodine, Iron, Manganese, Molybdenum, Nickel, Silicon, Vanadium, and Zinc.* Washington, DC: National Academy Press; 2001.

52. Institute of Medicine. *Dietary Reference Intakes for Calcium, Phosphorus, Magnesium, Vitamin D, and Fluoride.* Washington, DC: National Academy Press; 1997.

53. Institute of Medicine. *Dietary Reference Intakes for Vitamin C, Vitamin E, Selenium, and Carotenoids.* Washington, DC: National Academy Press; 2000.

54. Institute of Medicine. *Dietary Reference Intakes for Thiamin, Riboflavin, Niacin, Vitamin B6, Folate, Vitamin B12, Pantothenic Acid, Biotin, and Choline.* Washington, DC: National Academy Press; 2000.

55. Institute of Medicine. *Nutrition During Lactation.* Washington DC: National Academy Press; 1991.

56. Albareda M, Caballero A, Badell G, Piquer S, Ortiz A, De Leiva A, Corcoy R. Diabetes and abnormal glucose tolerance in women with previous gestational diabetes. *Diabetes Care.* 2003; 26:1199–1205.

57. Lauenborg J, Hansen T, Moller Jensen D, Vestergaard H, Molsted-Pedersen L, Hornnes P, Locht H, Pederson O, Damm P. Increasing incidence of diabetes after gestational diabetes. *Diabetes Care.* 2004;27:1194–1199.

58. Damm P, Kuhl C, Bertelsen A, Molsted-Pedersen L. Predictive factors for the development of diabetes in women with previous gestational diabetes mellitus. *Am J Obstet Gynecol.* 1992; 167:607–616.

59. Buchanan TA, Xiang A, Kjos SL, Lee WP, Trigo E, Nade N, Bergner A, Palmer J, Peters RK. Gestational diabetes: antepartum characteristics that predict postpartum glucose intolerance and type 2 diabetes in Latino women. *Diabetes.* 1998;47:1302–1310.

60. Jovanovic L, ed. *Medical Management of Pregnancy Complicated by Diabetes.* 3rd ed. Alexandria, Va: American Diabetes Association; 2000.

61. Rates and risk factors for recurrence of gestational diabetes. *Diabetes Care.* 2001;24:659–662.

62. Moses RG, Shand JL, Tapsell LC. The recurrence of gestational diabetes: could dietary differences in fat intake be an explanation? *Diabetes Care.* 1997;20:1647–1650.

63. Lu GC, Luchesse A, Chapman V, Cliver S, Rouse DJ. Screening for gestational diabetes mellitus in the subsequent pregnancy: is it worthwhile? *Am J Obstet Gynecol.* 2002;187:918–921.

64. Pallardo LF, Herranz L, Martin-Vaquero P, Garcia-Ingelmo T, Grande C, Janez M. Impaired fasting glucose and impaired glucose tolerance in women with prior gestational diabetes are associated with a different cardiovascular profile. *Diabetes Care.* 2003;26:2318–2322.

65. Zemel MB, Thompson W, Milstead A, Morris K, Campbell P. Calcium and dairy acceleration of weight and fat loss during energy restriction in obese adults. *Obes Res.* 2004;12:582–590.

66. Kaiser LL, Allen L; American Dietetic Association. Position of the American Dietetic Association: nutrition and lifestyle for a healthy pregnancy outcome. *J Am Diet Assoc.* 2002;102:1479–1490.

67. Landon MB, Gabbe SG. Diabetes mellitus. In: Barron WM, Lindheimer MD, eds. *Medical Disorders in Pregnancy.* 3rd ed. St. Louis, Mo: Mosby; 2000:71–100.

68. Kjos SL, Peters RK, Xiang A, Thomas D, Schaefer U, Buchanan TA. Contraception and the risk of type 2 diabetes mellitus in Latina women with prior gestational diabetes mellitus. *JAMA.* 1998;280:533–538.

69. Kjos SL. Contraception in diabetic women. *Obstet Gynecol Clin North Am.* 1996;23:243–258.

70. Landon MB, Catalano PM, Gabbe SG. Diabetes mellitus. In: Gabbe SG, Niebyl JR, Simpson JL, eds. *Obstetrics: Normal and Problem Pregnancies.* 4th ed. New York, NY: Churchill Livingstone; 2002:1081–1116.

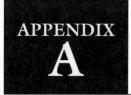

Forms

Referral Form to Health Care Provider

Name of Patient:_____ Date:_____

Address:_____

Tel. No:_____ Fax No:_____ E-mail:_____

Name of Insurance Co:_____

Tel. No:_____ Authorization No:_____

Age:_____ Gravida:_____ Para:_____ Ab/Misc:_____ EDC:_____

Height:_____ Current weight:_____ Prepregnancy weight:_____ Usual weight:_____

Medical History

Present history:_____

Past medical history:_____

Previous obstetric history:_____

Laboratory Data

Test:_____ Date:_____   Test: _____ Date: _____

Test:_____ Date:_____   Test: _____ Date: _____

Test:_____ Date:_____   Test: _____ Date: _____

Test:_____ Date:_____   Test: _____ Date: _____

Test:_____ Date:_____   Test: _____ Date: _____

Self-monitoring blood glucose? Yes _____ No _____

Medications

Please specify: _____

Reason for referral:_____

Signature of Health Care Provider: _____

Name of Health Care Provider: (please print)_____

Tel No:_____ Fax No:_____

I authorize for the following medical information to be released to:_____

Signature of patient:_____

Nutrition Questionnaire

Name:_____ Date:_____

Age:_____ Estimated due date:_____

Present weight:_____ Height:_____ Weight prior to this pregnancy:_____

Please answer the following questions:

How would you describe your appetite?　( ) Good　　( ) Fair　　( ) Poor

Have your eating habits changed with this pregnancy?　( ) Yes　　( ) No

    If yes, list changes_____

Are you following any diets/food plans?

Weight Loss	( ) Yes	( ) No	Low Fat/Low Cholesterol	( ) Yes	( ) No	
Diabetes	( ) Yes	( ) No	Low Sodium/No Salt	( ) Yes	( ) No	
Other	( ) Yes	( ) No				

    If yes, describe_____

Have you experienced any of these symptoms during your pregnancy?

Nausea	( ) Yes	( ) No	Heartburn	( ) Yes	( ) No
Vomiting	( ) Yes	( ) No	Hemorrhoids	( ) Yes	( ) No
Diarrhea	( ) Yes	( ) No	Excessive Saliva	( ) Yes	( ) No
Constipation	( ) Yes	( ) No	Dental Problems/	( ) Yes	( ) No
Other Illness	( ) Yes	( ) No	Bleeding Gums		

Are you experiencing any symptoms now?　( ) Yes　　( ) No

    If yes, please list_____

Are you a vegetarian?　( ) Yes　　( ) No　　If yes, do you eat any of the following?

Eggs	( ) Yes	( ) No	Cheese	( ) Yes	( ) No
Yogurt	( ) Yes	( ) No	Milk	( ) Yes	( ) No
Poultry	( ) Yes	( ) No	Fish	( ) Yes	( ) No

Do you eat raw meat, raw fish, raw eggs, or unpasteurized milk?　( ) Yes　　( ) No

List any food allergies or food intolerance:_____

Are there foods you cannot eat?_____
If so, why? _____

Do you eat any of the following?

Corn Starch	( ) Yes	( ) No	Ice	( ) Yes	( ) No
Laundry Starch	( ) Yes	( ) No	Clay	( ) Yes	( ) No
Dirt	( ) Yes	( ) No	Plaster	( ) Yes	( ) No
Paint Chips	( ) Yes	( ) No	Other Cravings	( ) Yes	( ) No	If yes, please list: _____

Are you taking any of the following?

Prenatal vitamin/mineral supplement　　( ) Yes　　( ) No

    Name:_____

Other vitamin/mineral supplement　　( ) Yes　　( ) No

    Name:_____

Iron supplement   ( ) Yes   ( ) No
     Name:_____

Herbal medication/supplement   ( ) Yes   ( ) No
     Name:_____

Laxatives   ( ) Yes   ( ) No
     Name:_____

Antacids   ( ) Yes   ( ) No
     Name:_____

Other over-the-counter medicines   ( ) Yes   ( ) No
     Name:_____

Prescription medicines   ( ) Yes   ( ) No
     Name:_____

Other medicines   ( ) Yes   ( ) No
     Name:_____

"Street" Drugs   ( ) Yes   ( ) No
     Name:_____

Are you taking insulin?   ( ) Yes   ( ) No
     If yes, list names and amount: _____

Are you testing your blood sugar/glucose?   ( ) Yes   ( ) No
     If yes, when do you test? _____

How much did you smoke before you were pregnant?
Do not smoke ( )   Less than 10/day ( )   10–20/day ( )   More than 20/day ( )

How much do you smoke now?
Do not smoke ( )   Less than 10/day ( )   10–20/day ( )   More than 20/day ( )

How often do you drink any of the following: beer, wine, wine coolers, hard liquor, mixed drinks, malt liquor?
Daily ( )   Weekly ( )   Monthly ( )   Never ( )

How many drinks do you have?   0 ( )   1 ( )   2 ( )   3 ( )   More ( )
Do you cook with alcohol?   ( ) Yes   ( ) No

Who does the cooking? _____ Who does the food shopping? _____

How often do you eat out? _____

Do you avoid eating any foods because of cultural or religious practice?   ( ) Yes   ( ) No
If yes, specify_____

Are you on WIC?   ( ) Yes   ( ) No
Do you receive Food Stamps?   ( ) Yes   ( ) No

How do you plan to feed your baby?   Breastmilk ( )   Formula ( )   Both ( )   Undecided ( )

Have you breastfed previously?   ( ) Yes   ( ) No
     If yes, how long did you breastfeed? _____

How often do you exercise? _____
List types of exercises: _____

Type of work/school:_____
If work, number of hours:_____
If school, present grade:_____

24-Hour Food Recall

Name: _____   Date: _____

Please write down everything you ate and drank yesterday from the time you woke up until the time you went to bed. Include all meals, snacks, and beverages and if you ate during the night.

Time	Type of Food or Beverage	Amount

Is this the way you usually eat? If not, what is the difference? _____

_____

_____

Food Frequency Questionnaire

Name:_____ Date:_____

Please indicate the number of times per day you eat the foods/beverages in each group. Circle the foods or beverages within each group.

Food	Daily	Weekly	Monthly	Barely or Never
Milk (whole, 2%, 1%, skim, buttermilk, chocolate, evaporated)				
Cheese (type)_____				
Ice cream, yogurt, pudding, flan				
Meat, poultry, or fish: Hamburger, roast beef, steak, pork chops, ham, chicken, turkey, ribs, fish, shell fish, lamb, tuna fish, liver, other_____				
Cold cuts, luncheon meats, hot dogs, sausages, bacon, canned meat				
Eggs				
Casseroles, stews, macaroni and cheese, chili, pizza, lasagna, tacos				
Dried beans, nuts, peanut butter				
Dark green, yellow, or orange vegetables: Broccoli, greens (collards, beets, turnip, kale, swiss chard, mustard), carrots, spinach, plantain, yams, sweet potato, squash, pumpkin, calabaza				
Other vegetables: Peas, string beans, potatoes, corn, mixed vegetables, beets, okra, eggplant, yucca, other_____				
Vitamin C fruits and/or juices: Orange, grapefruit, tomato, strawberries, pineapple				
Other fruits and/or juices: Apples, bananas, papaya, mango, peaches, pears, nectarines, honeydew, watermelon, cherries, grapes, other_____				
Cereal (cooked or ready-to-eat) _____				

Food	Daily	Weekly	Monthly	Barely or Never
Rice, noodles, macaroni, spaghetti, soup				
Bread (white, whole-wheat, rye), toast, crackers, rolls, cornbread, biscuits, bagels, tortillas, pancakes, pita, waffles, muffins				
Fruit drinks: Kool-Aid, Hi-C, Tang, Hawaiian Punch, lemonade, Sunny Delight, Malta, other _____				
Soda, coffee, tea (iced or hot)				
Candy, cake, cookies, pastries, doughnuts, gelatin desserts				
Potato chips, tortilla chips, corn chips, popcorn, pretzels				
Butter, margarine, salad dressing, mayonnaise, gravy, sour cream, cream cheese, oil				
Jams, jellies, marmalade, honey, syrup, sugar				
Water				
Beer, wine, wine coolers, hard liquor, malt liquor				
Fast foods (eg, french fries)				
Other_____				

Nutrition Assessment Form and Care Plan

Name: _____ Date: _____ Age: _____ EDC: _____

Subjective

Medical history: _____

Obstetric history: _____

Smoking: _____ Alcohol: _____ Substance use: _____

Medications: _____

Appetite/Recent changes: _____

GI discomforts: _____ Allergies/Intolerance: _____

Pica/Cravings/Aversions: _____ Food preferences: _____

Occupation/Educational level: _____ Hours worked/school: _____

Cultural/religious influences: _____ Language: _____

Food Assistance (Food Stamps, WIC): _____ Financial situation: _____

Lives with: _____ Food preparer/purchaser: _____

Exercise: _____ Exercise restrictions: _____

Insulin therapy:_____

SMBG—Frequency: _____ Testing times: _____ Type of meter: _____

Infant feeding plans: Breast: _____ Bottle: _____ Undecided: _____

Objective

Gravida: _____ Para: _____ AB/Misc: _____ Week of gestation: _____

Wt: _____ Ht: _____ Prepregnancy wt: _____ BMI: _____ Desirable wt: _____

Total wt gain: _____ Wt gain goals: _____

Lab Data: B/P: _____ Date: _____ Hgb/Hct: _____ Date: _____

Urine ketones: _____ Date: _____ OGCT: _____ Date: _____

OGTT: _____ Date: _____

Source: Adapted with permission from *American Dietetic Association Medical Nutrition Therapy Evidence-Based Guides for Practice: Nutrition Practice Guidelines for Gestational Diabetes Mellitus* [CD-ROM]. Chicago, Ill: American Dietetic Association; 2001.

Food Plan Calculations

Visit No.:_____   Date:_____

Food Group	B	S	L	S	D	S	S	Total Servings	Carbohydrate, g	Protein, g	Fat, g	Energy, kcal
Starch												
Fruit												
Milk												
Vegetables												
Meat												
Fat												

Total energy intake   = _____ kcal

Total carbohydrate   _____ × 4 = _____   % kcal _____

Total protein   _____ × 4 = _____   % kcal _____

Total fat   _____ × 9 = _____   % kcal _____

Requirements: Energy_____   Carbohydrate _____   Protein _____   Fat_____

Name of Person Completing Form:_____

Source: Adapted with permission from *American Dietetic Association Medical Nutrition Therapy Evidence-Based Guides for Practice: Nutrition Practice Guidelines for Gestational Diabetes Mellitus* [CD-ROM]. Chicago, Ill: American Dietetic Association; 2001.

Gestational Diabetes Blood Glucose and Food Record Form

Visit_____

Write down everything you eat, including the amounts and how the food was prepared.

Blood Test	Food/How Prepared	Amount	OFFICE USE ONLY					
			Carb					
			Starch	Fruit	Milk	Veg	Meat	Fat
Fasting: _____	**Breakfast:** Time:							
After breakfast: _____	**Snack:** Time:							
After lunch: _____	**Lunch:** Time:							
	Snack: Time:							
After dinner: _____	**Dinner:** Time:							
	Snack: Time:							
		Total						

Medical Nutrition Therapy Progress Notes: Gestational Diabetes Mellitus

Client Name: _____   Phone No.: _____

Medical record No.: _____   DOB: _____

Ethnic background: _____   Referring physician: _____

Outcomes of Medical Nutrition Therapy (MNT)

Expected Outcome	Intervention provided to meet goal (Intervention = self-management training plus client verbalizes/demonstrates)				Goal reached (Check indicates outcome achieved, follow with number 1–5 as indicated * e.g. ✓-3, ✓-5)							
Encounters	1	2	3	4**	Date 1	___ min	Date 2	___ min	Date 3	___ min	Date 4	___ min
					Value		Value		Value		Value	
Clinical Outcomes												
• Fasting blood glucose (*mean*)					___		___		___		___	
• 1-hour postpartum blood glucose (*mean*)					___		___		___		___	
• 2-hour postpartum blood glucose (*mean*)					___		___		___		___	
• Urine/blood ketones					___		___		___		___	
• A1C					___		___		___		___	
• Blood pressure					___		___		___		___	
• Weight					___		___		___		___	
MNT Goal: _____ kcal _____ g CARB — Adheres to appropriate meal, exercise, and medication treatment plan, to maintain blood glucose within normal limits and to have appropriate weight gain.					___ kcal ___ g CARB ___ meals ___ snacks		___ kcal ___ g CARB ___ meals ___ snacks		___ kcal ___ g CARB ___ meals ___ snacks		___ kcal ___ g CARB ___ meals ___ snacks	
Knowledge & Behavioral Outcomes*												
• Eats meals/snacks at consistent times					1 2 3 4 5		1 2 3 4 5		1 2 3 4 5		1 2 3 4 5	
• Chooses appropriate kinds/amounts of food					1 2 3 4 5		1 2 3 4 5		1 2 3 4 5		1 2 3 4 5	

• Demonstrates use of a meal planning system		1 2 3 4 5	1 2 3 4 5	1 2 3 4 5	1 2 3 4 5
• Recognizes foods that contain carbohydrate	1 2 3 4 5	1 2 3 4 5	1 2 3 4 5	1 2 3 4 5	1 2 3 4 5
• Reads food labels accurately	1 2 3 4 5	1 2 3 4 5	1 2 3 4 5	1 2 3 4 5	1 2 3 4 5
• States appropriate weight gain during pregnancy	1 2 3 4 5	1 2 3 4 5	1 2 3 4 5	1 2 3 4 5	1 2 3 4 5
• Tests blood glucose	___ x/day	___ x/day	___ x/day	___ x/day	___ x/day
• Records blood glucose daily	1 2 3 4 5	1 2 3 4 5	1 2 3 4 5	1 2 3 4 5	1 2 3 4 5
• Records food intake daily	1 2 3 4 5	1 2 3 4 5	1 2 3 4 5	1 2 3 4 5	1 2 3 4 5
• Verbalizes relationship of food, blood glucose, and physical activity	1 2 3 4 5	1 2 3 4 5	1 2 3 4 5	1 2 3 4 5	1 2 3 4 5
• Tests urine ketones	1 2 3 4 5	1 2 3 4 5	1 2 3 4 5	1 2 3 4 5	1 2 3 4 5
• Participates in regular activity per exercise plan	___ x/wk	___ x/wk	___ x/wk	___ x/wk	___ x/wk
• Verbalizes understanding of treatment for hypoglycemia, sick days, and consistency of diet/insulin/physical activity (if on insulin)		1 2 3 4 5	1 2 3 4 5	1 2 3 4 5	1 2 3 4 5
• Takes prenatal vitamin/mineral supplement as prescribed	1 2 3 4 5	1 2 3 4 5	1 2 3 4 5	1 2 3 4 5	1 2 3 4 5
• Abstains from smoking/alcohol use	1 2 3 4 5	1 2 3 4 5	1 2 3 4 5	1 2 3 4 5	1 2 3 4 5
• Verbalizes benefit of breast-feeding	1 2 3 4 5	1 2 3 4 5	1 2 3 4 5	1 2 3 4 5	1 2 3 4 5
• Verbalizes strategies for preventing type 2 diabetes	1 2 3 4 5	1 2 3 4 5	1 2 3 4 5	1 2 3 4 5	1 2 3 4 5

*Overall Adherence Potential**

Comprehension	1 2 3 4 5	1 2 3 4 5	1 2 3 4 5	1 2 3 4 5	1 2 3 4 5
Receptivity (readiness)	1 2 3 4 5	1 2 3 4 5	1 2 3 4 5	1 2 3 4 5	1 2 3 4 5
Adherence	1 2 3 4 5	1 2 3 4 5	1 2 3 4 5	1 2 3 4 5	1 2 3 4 5

Intervention: D, discussed; R, reinforced/reviewed; ≠, not reviewed; ✓, outcome achieved *, N/A- Not applicable.

*Key for Compliance Potential and Overall Adherence Potential: 1 = Never demonstrated; 2 = Rarely demonstrated; 3 = Sometimes demonstrated; 4 = Often demonstrated; 5 = Consistently demonstrated.

**Reproduce progress notes for encounters 5-7.

INITIAL VISIT

Date: _____

Beginning Time: _____ Ending Time: _____ Total Minutes: _____

Comments: _____

_____

_____

Client Goals: _____

Material Provided: _____

RD Signature: _____

Next Visit: _____

FOLLOW-UP VISIT

Date: _____

Beginning Time: _____ Ending Time: _____ Total Minutes: _____

Comments: _____

_____

_____

Client Goals: _____

Material Provided: _____

RD Signature: _____

Next Visit: _____

FOLLOW-UP VISIT

Date: _____

Beginning Time: _____ Ending Time: _____ Total Minutes: _____

Comments: _____

_____

_____

Client Goals: _____

Material Provided: _____

Next Visit: _____   RD Signature: _____

FOLLOW-UP VISIT

Beginning Time: _____   Ending Time: _____   Date: _____   Total Minutes: _____

Comments: _____

_____

Client Goals: _____

Material Provided: _____

Next Visit: _____   RD Signature: _____

Source: Adapted with permission from *American Dietetic Association Medical Nutrition Therapy Evidence-Based Guides for Practice: Nutrition Practice Guidelines for Gestational Diabetes Mellitus* [CD-ROM]. Chicago, Ill: American Dietetic Association; 2001.

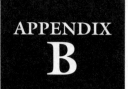

Case Studies

Alyce M. Thomas, RD, and Yolanda M. Gutierrez, MS, PhD, RD

INTRODUCTION

The following case studies are clinical applications of the concepts outlined in Chapter 6. These are only examples and are not strict guidelines for providing medical nutrition therapy (MNT). Registered dietitian (RD) protocol for treatment of gestational diabetes mellitus (GDM) may vary. For example, some RDs are limited to seeing their patients once. Other RDs do not have access to laboratory data. For the purposes of these studies, multiple visits and access to laboratory data are assumed. Documenting the care of the client at each visit is essential for verifying the quality and outcome of care (1). The RD documents the assessment data, intervention plan, patient goals, and recommendations in the medical record (1).

LACTOSE-INTOLERANT CLIENT WITH HIGH-RISK PREGNANCY

Visit 1

Client Data

Mariana is a 26-year-old woman from Mexico. She was referred from an obstetric clinic to a high-risk pregnancy center. Mariana (gravida 1, para 0) is at 22 weeks' gestation. She has a family history of diabetes mellitus (DM); her maternal grandmother was diagnosed with DM many years ago.

Mariana is a housewife and lives with her husband in a five-room, second-floor apartment. The pregnancy was unplanned, but both Mariana and her husband are happy. Mariana does not smoke, drink alcohol, or use drugs, but she is exposed to second-hand smoke. Mariana expresses concerns about her family's finances and the new baby because she is not working.

Mariana's education level is determined to be approximately tenth grade. She quit school in the tenth grade.

Mariana is five feet tall (60 inches) and weighs 175 lb. Her BMI is 34.2. Her prepregnancy weight was 166 lb. Because her pregnancy is high risk, her doctor has not medically cleared her to walk.

The laboratory values are blood pressure, 108/72 mm Hg; Hgb, 12.5 mg/dL; Hct, 36.5%; A1C, 6.0%; 1-hour glucose challenge test (GCT), 187 mg/dL; 3-hour oral glucose tolerance test (OGTT): fasting, 116 mg/dL; 1 hour, 182 mg/dL; 2 hour, 168 mg/dL; 3 hour, 126 mg/dL.

Assessment

The RD asks Mariana to complete the nutrition questionnaire, the food frequency form, and the 24-hour recall form (see Figures B.1, B.2, and B.3 [pp. 133–134, 135–136, 137]). Mariana explains that she is lactose intolerant but is able to tolerate cheese and small amounts of milk at breakfast. She does not like yogurt.

The dietitian completes the nutrition assessment and care plan and food calculation forms (Figures B.4 and B.5 [pp. 138, 139]). Mariana's estimated energy intake is 2,200 kcal/day. Her energy needs are 1,800 kcal/day.

In providing MNT, the RD explains that Mariana's blood glucose goals are <95 mg/dL (fasting) and <120 mg/dL (2 hours postprandial). The RD explains that Mariana needs to monitor her blood glucose four times daily (fasting and 2 hours postprandial).

Mariana is instructed and evaluated by a clinical nurse specialist. A fetal echocardiogram was performed, because Mariana may have had type 2 diabetes before pregnancy. A fetal echocardiogram is a specialized ultrasound that focuses on the fetal heart and is performed by a pediatric cardiologist.

Intervention

The RD creates an individualized 1,800-kcal meal plan:

- Breakfast: 2 carbohydrate, 1 meat, 1 fat
- Morning snack: 1 carbohydrate
- Lunch: 3 carbohydrate, 3 meats, 1 vegetable, 1 fat
- Afternoon snack: 1 carbohydrate
- Dinner: 4 carbohydrate, 3 meats, 2 vegetables, 1 fat
- Evening snack: 2 carbohydrate, 1 meat, 1 fat

The RD sets the following nutrition goals for Mariana:

- Decrease carbohydrate intake at breakfast to 30 g
- SMBG four times daily
- Eliminate fried foods
- Decrease juice intake
- Increase calcium intake to DRI of 1,200 mg, with cheese and calcium supplement
- Return in 1 week with blood glucose and food record form

The RD completes the MNT progress note (see pp. 126–129 in Appendix A for form).

Visit 2

Assessment

At visit 2, Mariana's first follow-up visit, she is at 24 weeks' gestation. Her weight is 178 lb, and her blood pressure is 121/66 mm Hg. Her test for ketones is negative.

Nutrition Questionnaire (Visit 1)

Name: _Mariana_ _____   Date: ___10/28/03_____

Age: __26_____   Estimated due date: __3/3/04_____

Present weight: __175____   Height: ___5'0"___   Weight prior to this pregnancy: ___166_____

Please answer the following questions:

How would you describe your appetite?   (X) Good   (   ) Fair   (   ) Poor

Have your eating habits changed with this pregnancy?   (   ) Yes   (X) No

    If yes, list changes_____

Are you following any diets/food plans?

Weight Loss	( ) Yes	(X) No	Low Fat/Low Cholesterol	( ) Yes	(X) No
Diabetes	(X) Yes	( ) No	Low Sodium/No Salt	( ) Yes	(X) No
Other	( ) Yes	(X) No			

    If yes, describe_____

Have you experienced any of these symptoms during your pregnancy?

Nausea	( ) Yes	(X) No	Heartburn	( ) Yes	(X) No
Vomiting	( ) Yes	(X) No	Hemorrhoids	( ) Yes	(X) No
Diarrhea	( ) Yes	(X) No	Excessive Saliva	( ) Yes	(X) No
Constipation	( ) Yes	(X) No	Dental Problems/	( ) Yes	(X) No
Other Illness	( ) Yes	(X) No	Bleeding Gums		

Are you experiencing any symptoms now?   (   ) Yes   (X) No

    If yes, please list_____

Are you a vegetarian?   (   ) Yes   (X) No   If yes, do you eat any of the following?

Eggs	( ) Yes	( ) No	Cheese	( ) Yes	( ) No
Yogurt	( ) Yes	( ) No	Milk	( ) Yes	( ) No
Poultry	( ) Yes	( ) No	Fish	( ) Yes	( ) No

Do you eat raw meat, raw fish, raw eggs, or unpasteurized milk?   (   ) Yes   (X) No

List any food allergies or food intolerance: ____Milk_____

Are there foods you cannot eat?____Yogurt_____

If so, why? ____Don't like the taste._____

Do you eat any of the following?

Corn Starch	( ) Yes	(X) No	Ice	( ) Yes	(X) No
Laundry Starch	( ) Yes	(X) No	Clay	( ) Yes	(X) No
Dirt	( ) Yes	(X) No	Plaster	( ) Yes	(X) No
Paint Chips	( ) Yes	(X) No	Other Cravings	( ) Yes	(X) No

If yes, please list: _____

Are you taking any of the following?

Prenatal vitamin/mineral supplement   (X) Yes   (   ) No

    Name:_____

Other vitamin/mineral supplement   (   ) Yes   (X) No

    Name:_____

FIGURE B.1.   Visit 1. Nutrition questionnaire.

Iron supplement ( ) Yes (X) No
Name:_____

Herbal medication/supplement ( ) Yes (X) No
Name:_____

Laxatives ( ) Yes (X) No
Name:_____

Antacids ( ) Yes (X) No
Name:_____

Other over-the-counter medicines ( ) Yes (X) No
Name:_____

Prescription medicines ( ) Yes (X) No
Name:_____

Other medicines ( ) Yes (X) No
Name:_____

"Street" Drugs ( ) Yes (X) No
Name:_____

Are you taking insulin? ( ) Yes (X) No
If yes, list names and amount: _____

Are you testing your blood sugar/glucose? ( ) Yes (X) No
If yes, when do you test? _____

How much did you smoke before you were pregnant?
Do not smoke (X) Less than 10/day ( ) 10–20/day ( ) More than 20/day ( )

How much do you smoke now?
Do not smoke (X) Less than 10/day ( ) 10–20/day ( ) More than 20/day ( )

How often do you drink any of the following: beer, wine, wine coolers, hard liquor, mixed drinks, malt liquor?
Daily ( ) Weekly ( ) Monthly ( ) Never (X)

How many drinks do you have? 0 (X) 1 ( ) 2 ( ) 3 ( ) More ( )
Do you cook with alcohol? ( ) Yes (X) No

Who does the cooking? ____Me____ Who does the food shopping? ____Me____

How often do you eat out? ____Once a week____

Do you avoid eating any foods because of cultural or religious practice? ( ) Yes (X) No
If yes, specify_____

Are you on WIC? (X) Yes ( ) No
Do you receive Food Stamps? (X) Yes ( ) No

How do you plan to feed your baby? Breastmilk (X) Formula ( ) Both ( ) Undecided ( )

Have you breastfed previously? ( ) Yes ( ) No
If yes, how long did you breastfeed? _____

How often do you exercise? ____No, doctor tells me not to____
List types of exercises: _____

Type of work/school:____Stay-at-home mom____
If work, number of hours:_____
If school, present grade:____Dropped out of school in 10th grade____

FIGURE B.1. (*continued*)

Food Frequency Questionnaire

Name:_____Mariana_____ Date:_____10/28/03_____

Please indicate the number of times per day you eat the foods/beverages in each group. Circle the foods or beverages within each group.

Food	Daily	Weekly	Monthly	Barely or Never
Milk ((whole), 2%, 1%, skim, buttermilk, chocolate, evaporated)				0
Cheese (type)_ white, American sliced _____		4		
Ice cream, yogurt, pudding,(flan)			1	
Meat, poultry, or fish: (Hamburger), roast beef,(steak),(pork chops),(ham,) (chicken), turkey, ribs, fish, shell fish, lamb,(tuna fish), liver, other_____	1			
Cold cuts, luncheon meats, hot dogs,(sausages), bacon, (canned meat)		5		
Eggs		3		
Casseroles, stews, macaroni and cheese, chili,(pizza,) lasagna,(tacos)		2		
(Dried beans,) nuts, peanut butter		3		
Dark green, yellow, or orange vegetables: (Broccoli,) greens (collards, beets, turnip, kale, swiss chard, mustard), carrots,(spinach)(plantain,) yams, sweet potato, squash, pumpkin, calabaza		5		
Other vegetables: Peas, string beans,(potatoes,)(corn,) mixed vegetables,(beets,) okra, eggplant, yucca, other_____		4		
Vitamin C fruits and/or juices: (Orange,) grapefruit, tomato, strawberries, pineapple	2			
Other fruits and/or juices: (Apples,)(bananas,) papaya, (mango,) peaches, pears, nectarines, honeydew,(watermelon,) cherries, grapes, other_____	2			
Cereal (cooked or ready-to-eat) __Cornflakes_____		2		

FIGURE B.2. Visit 1. Food frequency questionnaire.

Food	Daily	Weekly	Monthly	Barely or Never
(Rice), noodles, macaroni, (spaghetti) (soup)		5		
Bread ((white) whole-wheat, rye), toast, (crackers), rolls, cornbread, biscuits, bagels, (tortillas), pancakes, pita, waffles, muffins	4			
Fruit drinks: Kool-Aid, Hi-C, Tang, Hawaiian Punch, lemonade, Sunny Delight, Malta, other _____				0
(Soda), coffee, tea (iced or hot)	1			
Candy, (cake) (cookies), pastries, doughnuts, gelatin desserts		3		
Potato chips, (tortilla chips), corn chips, popcorn, pretzels			2	
(Butter), margarine, salad dressing, (mayonnaise), gravy, (sour cream), cream cheese, (oil)	3			
Jams, jellies, marmalade, honey, syrup, (sugar)	1			
Water	2			
Beer, wine, wine coolers, hard liquor, malt liquor				0
Fast foods (eg, french fries)			1	

FIGURE B.2. (*continued*)

Estimated fetal weight by ultrasonography at 22 weeks and 4 days gestation is 492 g. The measurements of the fetus are consistent.

Mariana has completed the blood glucose and food record form (Figure B.6), which shows that her fasting blood glucose is 87–112 mg/dL and her 2-hour postprandial blood glucose is 50–196 mg/dL. Mariana was admitted to the antepartum unit for insulin initiation. Her insulin plan consists of 46 units (30 units NPH, 16 units regular) in the morning, 16 units (regular) in the afternoon, and 10 units (NPH) in the evening.

Mariana complains of hunger with the meal plan. She has increased her breakfast carbohydrate intake to 3, lunch carbohydrate to 7, and dinner carbohydrate to 5. She did not have a meat choice for the evening snack. Mariana explains that she occasionally eats home-made chicken soup for breakfast.

The RD completes the food plan calculation form (Figure B.7 [p. 141]) and notes that Mariana is not taking a calcium supplement.

24-Hour Food Recall

Name: _____Mariana_____ Date: __11/20/03_____

Please write down everything you ate and drank yesterday from the time you woke up until the time you went to bed. Include all meals, snacks, and beverages and if you ate during the night.

Time	Type of Food or Beverage	Amount
8:00 am	Cereal	1 small bowl
	Milk	8 ounces
	Apple	1 small
10:00 am	Banana	1 small
	Orange juice	8 ounces
1:00 pm	Fried Chicken	2 legs
	Salad with oil, vinegar, and lemon	2 cups
	Tortillas	4
3:30 pm	Orange juice	8 ounces
6:30 pm	Leftovers from lunch	
	Fried chicken	2 legs
	Salad with oil, vinegar, and lemon	2 cups
	Tortillas	4
9:00 pm	Apple	1 small

Is this the way you usually eat? If not, what is the difference? _____Yes_____

_____

_____

FIGURE B.3. Visit 1. 24-hour food recall.

Nutrition Assessment Form and Care Plan

Name: ___Mariana___ Date: ___10/28/03___ Age: ___26___ EDC: ___3/21/04___

Subjective

Medical history: ___Family history of diabetes___

Obstetric history: ___First pregnancy___

Smoking: ___No___ Alcohol: ___No___ Substance use: ___No, but exposed to second-hand smoke___

Medications: ___Prenatal vitamin/mineral supplement 1/day___

Appetite/Recent changes: ___Appetite is good; no recent changes in eating habits___

GI discomforts: ___None___ Allergies/Intolerance: ___None___

Pica/Cravings/Aversions: ___None___ Food preferences: ___Chicken soup___

Occupation/Educational level: ___Housewife, 10th-grade education___ Hours worked/school: ___N/A___

Cultural/religious influences: ___Hispanic___ Language ___Spanish___

Food Assistance (Food Stamps, WIC): ___WIC___ Financial situation: ___Husband works part-time in restaurant___

Lives with: ___Husband___ Food preparer/purchaser: ___Client___

Exercise: ___None___ Exercise restrictions: ___Not medically cleared___

Insulin therapy: ___Morning: 30 units NPH, 16 units Regular; Before dinner: 16 units Regular; Bedtime: 10 units NPH___

SMBG—Frequency: _4/day_ Testing times: ___FBG & 2-hour postmeal___ Type of meter: ___One Touch___

Infant feeding plans: Breast: ___X___ Bottle: _____ Undecided: _____

Objective

Gravida: ___1___ Para: ___0___ AB/Misc: ___0___ Week of gestation: ___22___

Wt: ___175 lb___ Ht: ___60 in___ Prepregnancy wt: ___166 lb___ BMI: ___34.2___ Desirable wt: ___115 lb___

Total wt gain: ___9 lb___ Wt gain goals: ___15 lb___

Lab Data: B/P: ___108/72 mm Hg___ Date: ___11/23/03___ Hgb/Hct: ___12.5/36.5___ Date: ___10/28/03___

Urine ketones: ___Neg.___ Date: ___10/28/03___ GCT: ___187 mg/dL___ Date: ___10/28/03___

OGTT: ___116/182/168/126___ Date: ___10/28/03___

FIGURE B.4. Visit 1. Nutrition assessment form and care plan. Form adapted with permission from: *American Dietetic Association Medical Nutrition Therapy Evidence-Based Guides for Practice: Nutrition Practice Guidelines for Gestational Diabetes Mellitus* [CD-ROM]. Chicago, Ill: American Dietetic Association; 2001.

Food Plan Calculations

Visit No.: __1__   Date: __10/28/03__

Food Group	B	S	L	S	D	S	S	Total Servings	Carbohydrate, g	Protein, g	Fat, g	Energy, kcal
Starch	1		4		4			9	105	27	5	720
Fruit	1	3		2			1	5	75			300
Milk	1							1	12	8	8	150
Vegetables		1		1				2	10	4		50
Meat		4		4				8		56	64	800
Fat		2		2				4			20	180

Total energy intake   = __2,200__ kcal

Total carbohydrate   __202__ × 4 = __808__   % kcal __37__

Total protein   __95__ × 4 = __380__   % kcal __17__

Total fat   __98__ × 9 = __882__   % kcal __40__

Requirements: Energy __1,800 kcal__   Carbohydrate __202 g__   Protein __90 g__   Fat __70 g__

Name of Person Completing Form: __Karen Adams, MS, RD, CDE__

FIGURE B.5. Visit 1. Food plan calculations. Form adapted with permission from: *American Dietetic Association Medical Nutrition Therapy Evidence-Based Guides for Practice: Nutrition Practice Guidelines for Gestational Diabetes Mellitus* [CD-ROM]. Chicago, Ill: American Dietetic Association; 2001.

Intervention

The RD adjusts the meal plan to decrease fat intake. Mariana's new energy intake is 1,900 kcal/day.

The RD explains why adequate calcium is important during pregnancy. The RD emphasizes that Mariana plan her meal and snack times with consistency. Mariana's goals are as follows:

- Add snacks to avoid consuming additional calories at meals
- Begin taking calcium supplement daily
- Decrease fat intake

Visit 3

Assessment

At Mariana's third visit with the RD, she is at 26 weeks' gestation and her weight has increased by 2 lb (body weight = 180 lb). Her blood pressure is 106/61 mm Hg. The test for

Gestational Diabetes Blood Glucose and Food Record Form

Visit __2__

Write down everything you eat, including the amounts and how the food was prepared.

Blood Test	Food/How Prepared	Amount	OFFICE USE ONLY					
			Carb					
			Starch	Fruit	Milk	Veg	Meat	Fat
Fasting: __102__	**Breakfast:** Tortillas Eggs (scrambled) Cheese (added to eggs) Butter Orange juice mixed with water **Time:** 7:30 am	2 2 1 slice 2 tsp 4 oz	2	1			3	2
After breakfast: _____	**Snack:** None **Time:**							
After lunch: __125__	**Lunch:** Tortillas Beans (refried) Lettuce Tomato Iced tea (made with sugar substitute **Time:** 12:30 pm	4 1 cup 1 small 12 oz	6			1	2	2
	Snack: Banana **Time:** 3:30 pm	1 small		1				
After dinner: __150__	**Dinner:** Chicken soup (made with noodles and vegetables) Rice Orange **Time:** 6:00 pm	2 bowls 1 cup 1	5	1		2	6	2
	Snack: None **Time:**							
	Total		13	3	0	3	11	6

FIGURE B.6. Visit 2. Gestational diabetes blood glucose and food record form.

Food Plan Calculations

Visit No.: __2__   Date: __11/27/03__

Food Group	B	S	L	S	D	S	S	Total Servings	Carbohydrate, g	Protein, g	Fat, g	Energy, kcal
Starch	2		6		5			13	195	9	5	1200
Fruit	1			1	1			3	45			180
Milk								0				
Vegetables			1		2			3	15	6		75
Meat	3		2		6			11		77	61	565
Fat	2		2		2			6			30	270

Total energy intake   = __2,290__ kcal

Total carbohydrate   __245__ × 4 = __980__   % kcal __43__

Total protein   __92__ × 4 = __368__   % kcal __16__

Total fat   __96__ × 9 = __864__   % kcal __38__

Requirements: Energy __1,900 kcal__   Carbohydrate __214 g__   Protein __95 g__   Fat __74 g__

Name of Person Completing Form: __Karen Adams, MS, RD, CDE__

FIGURE B.7.   Visit 2. Food plan calculation form. Form adapted with permission from: *American Dietetic Association Medical Nutrition Therapy Evidence-Based Guides for Practice: Nutrition Practice Guidelines for Gestational Diabetes Mellitus* [CD-ROM]. Chicago, Ill: American Dietetic Association; 2001.

ketones is negative. Mariana's blood glucose levels are improving (fasting: 91–103 mg/dL; 2 hours postprandial: 68–149 mg/dL) but continue to be above the optimal level.

Mariana complains of hunger just before meals. She drinks a large glass of water before eating, then has stomach pains after eating. The RD uses the Food Plan Calculation Form (Figure B.8 [p. 142]) to determine the adequacy of Mariana's eating habits. To keep her blood glucose levels within the normal range, she has eliminated her morning and afternoon snacks. She is compliant with the calcium supplement. The clinical nurse specialist reviews the insulin injection technique. The insulin plan is increased to 40 units NPH in the morning, 20 units regular insulin before breakfast, and 20 units regular insulin before dinner.

Intervention

Mariana will continue to monitor her blood glucose levels and measure her food for portion accuracy. The next appointment with the RD is scheduled in 2 weeks. Mariana is encouraged to attend her prenatal visits.

Food Plan Calculations

Visit No.:___3___   Date:___12/14/03___

Food Group	B	S	L	S	D	S	S	Total Servings	Carbohydrate, g	Protein, g	Fat, g	Energy, kcal
Starch	2		2		3		1	8	120	24	3	640
Fruit			1					1	15			60
Milk								0				
Vegetables					2			2	10	4		50
Meat	3		3		6		1	13		91	65	975
Fat			1					1			5	45

Total energy intake   = _1,170_ kcal

Total carbohydrate   _145_ × 4 = _580_   % kcal _33_

Total protein   _119_ × 4 = _476_   % kcal _27_

Total fat   _73_ × 9 = _657_   % kcal _37_

Requirements: Energy _1,900 kcal_   Carbohydrate _214 g_   Protein _95 g_   Fat _74 g_

Name of Person Completing Form:_ Karen Adams, MS, RD, CDE _

FIGURE B.8.   Visit 3. Food plan calculation form. Form adapted with permission from: *American Dietetic Association Medical Nutrition Therapy Evidence-Based Guides for Practice: Nutrition Practice Guidelines for Gestational Diabetes Mellitus* [CD-ROM]. Chicago, Ill: American Dietetic Association; 2001.

Visit 4

Assessment

Mariana is now 31 weeks pregnant, having missed three appointments. She weighs 186 lb, her blood pressure is 112/68 mm Hg, and she is negative for ketones. Mariana's fasting blood glucose is 85–100 mg/dL, and her 2-hour postprandial blood glucose is 103–136 mg/dL. Her amniotic fluid index is 19.7, and a nonstress test was reactive.

Mariana was referred to the social worker because of missed prenatal visits, although she has not missed her ultrasonography and biophysical profile appointments. She is no longer complaining of hunger and is compliant with the food plan. The RD uses the Food Plan Calculation Form (Figure B.9 [p. 143]) to determine the adequacy of Mariana's food plan. After the consultation with the social worker, Mariana states that she feels better and will continue with her insulin and blood glucose monitoring plan. Her insulin plan is increased by 2 units before breakfast and dinner (to 42 units of NPH and 22 units of regular before breakfast, and 22 units of regular before dinner); her evening insulin dose is not changed.

Food Plan Calculations

Visit No.: ___4___   Date: ___1/20/04___

Food Group	B	S	L	S	D	S	S	Total Servings	Carbohydrate, g	Protein, g	Fat, g	Energy, kcal
Starch	2	1	3		3		2	11	165	33	5	880
Fruit		1		1				2	30			120
Milk								0				
Vegetables			2		1			3	15	6		75
Meat	2	1	6		5		1	14		98	72	1,150
Fat	2		1					3			15	135

Total energy intake   = _2,360_ kcal

Total carbohydrate   _210_ × 4 = _980_   % kcal _42_

Total protein   _137_ × 4 = _548_   % kcal _23_

Total fat   _92_ × 9 = _828_   % kcal _35_

Requirements: Energy _1,900 kcal_   Carbohydrate _214 g_   Protein _95 g_   Fat _74 g_

Name of Person Completing Form: _Karen Adams, MS, RD, CDE_

FIGURE B.9.   Visit 4. Food plan calculation form. Form adapted with permission from: *American Dietetic Association Medical Nutrition Therapy Evidence-Based Guides for Practice: Nutrition Practice Guidelines for Gestational Diabetes Mellitus* [CD-ROM]. Chicago, Ill: American Dietetic Association; 2001.

Intervention

The RD reinforces the positive changes in Mariana's food plan. Additional food preferences are incorporated into her food plan using carbohydrate counting. As this is the last appointment with the RD, Mariana will continue her present insulin, food, and SMBG plan. The RD documents the visit in Mariana's medical records.

OBESE ADOLESCENT CLIENT

Visit 1

Client Data

Deborah is an 18-year-old white female referred from a teen obstetrical program at 22 weeks' gestation because of an abnormal oral glucose tolerance test (OGTT). She is gravida 2, para 0, with a previous spontaneous abortion at 12 weeks' gestation 1 year ago. She was diagnosed with hyperthyroidism before this pregnancy and is on synthroid.

Deborah has a family history of diabetes (mother and paternal grandmother). An early glucose screen is performed because of her family history. She is not experiencing any gastrointestinal discomforts except for occasional heartburn. She has expressed concern about gaining weight and the health of the fetus, because of the previous miscarriage. Deborah plans to breastfeed.

Deborah currently lives with her boyfriend in an attic apartment. She recently moved out of her parents' house because of family problems, about which she would not elaborate. She does not use alcohol or tobacco but occasionally smokes marijuana. She quit school in the 10th grade. Deborah has been medically cleared for low-impact exercises, such as walking.

Deborah is 5 feet, 6 inches tall, and weighs 220 lb. Her prepregnancy weight was 210 lb, with a BMI of 35. Her initial laboratory results are blood pressure, 121/68 mm Hg; Hgb, 11.4 mg/dL; Hct, 34.2%; A1C, 5.2%; GCT, 174 mg/dL; OGTT: fasting, 82 mg/dL; 1 hour, 171 mg/dL; 2 hour, 195 mg/dL; 3 hour, 173 mg/dL.

Assessment

The RD requests that Deborah complete the initial nutrition forms (nutrition questionnaire, 24-hour recall, and food frequency). The 24-hour recall is as follows:

- Breakfast (10:00 am): 2 eggs, 2 slices salami, 1 hash brown, 2 slices toast, 8 ounces orange juice
- Lunch: (3:00 pm): Egg salad sandwich made with 2 eggs, 2 slices bread, 1 tablespoon mayonnaise, can of soda
- Snack (3:30 pm): Bag of potato chips
- Dinner (7:30 pm): 2 fried chicken legs with 1 cup mashed potatoes and $^1/_2$ cup corn
- Snack (11:00 pm): Large bowl of frosted cereal with 1 cup regular milk

Deborah insists that she will not drink reduced-fat, low-fat, or nonfat milk. Her estimated energy intake is 2,520 kcal, and her estimated energy requirement is 2,200 kcal. On the advice of her obstetrician, Deborah is admitted for insulin initiation. Before admission, the blood glucose goals are explained (fasting: < 95 mg/dL; 1 hour postprandial: < 130 mg/dL). After discharge, she will monitor her blood glucose levels four times daily: fasting and 1 hour postmeals.

Intervention

Deborah is instructed on a 2,200-kcal food plan, consisting of 3 meals and 3 snacks per day. She is referred to the WIC Program and to a social worker because of her family situation. The following goals are set for Deborah:

- Keep her meal/snack times consistent
- Keep food records
- Strive for weight gain goals of $^2/_3$ lb/wk
- Begin walking program four times a week for 30 minutes
- Return in 1 week after hospital discharge

Visit 2

Assessment

Deborah is now at 23 weeks' gestation. Her weight is 220 lb, and her blood pressure is 121/73 mm Hg. She kept a food record for 2 days, but she has not followed the insulin plan from the hospital admission. The plan from the hospital consisted of three daily injections of short-acting and intermediate-acting insulin: 20 units NPH and 10 units regular insulin before breakfast, 10 units regular insulin before dinner, and 10 units insulin at bedtime. Deborah was injecting insulin twice daily: before breakfast and bedtime.

She was instructed on carbohydrate counting during her hospitalization but has difficulty understanding the concept. She has decreased her food intake to maintain normoglycemia. She is consistent with SMBG. Deborah has walked for 15 minutes only once since her initial visit and has stopped smoking marijuana.

Deborah's blood glucose ranges are as follows: fasting blood glucose, 72–100 mg/dL; 2 hours after breakfast, 85–158 mg/dL; 2 hours after lunch, 45–128 mg/dL; and 2 hours after dinner, 84–178 mg/dL. Her random blood glucose is 142 mg/dL.

Deborah's 2-day food record is as follows:

Day 1

- Breakfast (7:30 am): $1\frac{1}{2}$ cups unsweetened cereal with 1 cup whole milk
- Snack (10:30 am): Small orange
- Lunch (12:00 pm): 1 cup salad with 2 tablespoons ranch dressing and 1 dinner roll
- Snack (3:30 pm): 8 ounces low-fat yogurt and a bagel
- Dinner (6:30 pm): Baked chicken thighs (2) with 1 cup spaghetti with pasta sauce
- Snack (10:00 pm): $1\frac{1}{2}$ cups unsweetened cereal with 1 cup whole milk

Day 2

- Breakfast (8:00 am): Bagel with cream cheese
- Snack (10:30 am): Small orange
- Lunch (1:00 pm): Turkey and cheese sandwich (made with 2 slices turkey, 2 slices cheese, 2 slices bread, lettuce, 2 slices tomato, and 2 teaspoons mayonnaise)
- Snack (4:30 pm): 8 ounces low-fat yogurt and $\frac{1}{2}$ mango
- Dinner (6:00 pm): 1 pork chop, $\frac{1}{2}$ cup mashed potatoes, $\frac{1}{2}$ cup broccoli
- Snack (10:30 pm): $1\frac{1}{2}$ cups unsweetened cereal with 1 cup whole milk

Intervention

After reviewing Deborah's food and blood glucose records, the RD reinforces the importance of complying with the insulin plan. Carbohydrate counting is reviewed, and Deborah indicates that she understands the process. A protein source is added to breakfast, with emphasis on decreasing the carbohydrate intake at breakfast to two choices. Deborah is encouraged to include vegetables. Label reading, and fat and calcium intake are discussed.

Deborah's goals for her next visit are as follows:

- Follow insulin plan, as instructed by nurse educator
- Increase the frequency of walking to four times weekly
- Keep food record
- Continue SMBG four times daily
- Increase vegetable intake to at least three servings daily

Visit 3

Assessment

Deborah is now at 25 weeks' gestation and weighs 224 lb. Her blood pressure is 130/70 mm Hg. Her random blood glucose is 192 mg/dL, and she ate a croissant made with egg and cheese, and hash browns 1 hour before her appointment.

Deborah's fasting blood glucose is 79–91 mg/dL. Her 1-hour postprandial levels range from 69 to 137 mg/dL. Her health care provider increased the insulin plan by 2 units before breakfast and at dinner, but the bedtime insulin dosage was not changed.

Deborah walked 3 days for 20 minutes and kept both food and blood glucose records. She has eliminated fried foods and included a protein source at breakfast (egg or cheese or two thin slices of turkey). She is following her insulin plan correctly and has eliminated juice and prefers to eat fruit for morning and afternoon snacks.

Intervention

The RD emphasizes portion sizes, especially with carbohydrates, reviews label reading, and discusses incorporating convenience and fast foods into food plan.

Deborah's goals are as follows:

- Continue to keep food and blood glucose records
- Increase walking to 30 minutes
- Continue to increase vegetable intake

Visit 4

Assessment

Deborah is at 28 weeks' gestation. Her weight is 230 lb and her blood pressure is 115/65 mm Hg. Her random blood glucose is 105 mg/dL. Her blood glucose fasting levels were 63–99 mg/dL and her 1-hour postprandial values were 81–128 mg/dL.

Deborah is feeling better and is following the food plan. She is not experiencing any discomforts or hunger. Her walking program has increased to 35 minutes, 5 days per week. She is keeping food records and has eliminated fried foods. Deborah is following her insulin plan correctly. She has been compliant with increasing the protein intake at breakfast and with increasing her vegetable intake to at least three servings daily. She prefers to eat fruit for the morning and afternoon snacks and has eliminated juice.

Intervention

The RD encourages Deborah to continue the present regimen and discusses the rate of weight gain in the third trimester for her prepregnancy weight for height. Carbohydrate counting is reviewed. Deborah will do the following:

- Continue present food regimen of three meals and three snacks
- Continue appointments with RD every 2 weeks

Visit 5

Assessment

Deborah weighs 232 lb at 31 weeks' gestation and her blood pressure is 121/72 mm Hg. Her random blood glucose value is 111 mg/dL. Her fasting levels are 79–83 mg/dL and her 1-hour postprandial values are 92–121 mg/dL.

Deborah explains that she has been compliant with the food plan, exercise program, and insulin plan because she realizes that her blood glucose levels can affect the health of her baby. She has no complaints of hunger and is using carbohydrate counting because of its flexibility and the ability to eat a variety of foods.

Intervention

The RD discusses breastfeeding and postpartum nutrition issues with Deborah. Deborah will not be able to continue follow-up with the RD because of insurance coverage but will call if there are any issues.

Postpartum

Deborah calls the RD after delivery. She delivered at 39 weeks' gestation via cesarean section because labor would not progress. At birth, the infant weighed 3,365 g. Deborah is breastfeeding and following the postpartum food plan. She will have a 75-g OGTT at her 6-week postpartum check-up.

CLIENT WITH ADVANCED MATERNAL AGE, FIBROID UTERUS, LOW-CALORIE INTAKE

Visit 1

Elizabeth is a 40-year-old Haitian woman referred to a perinatologist at 15 weeks' gestation because of advanced maternal age, abnormal OGTT, fibroid uterus, and incompetent cervix with possible cerclage. She is gravida 2, para 1, and was referred for genetic counseling because of age. She declined amniocentesis. An early ultrasound confirmed pregnancy at 10 weeks and the presence of two fibroids. Elizabeth's family history reveals three sisters with type 2 diabetes. She is not experiencing gastrointestinal discomforts except for occasional constipation. Elizabeth does not smoke or drink. She plans to breastfeed.

Elizabeth lives with her husband and 11-year-old son. Her husband works part-time as a day laborer. She has completed high school. Although the pregnancy was unplanned, she has expressed willingness to continue the pregnancy. She does not have health insurance and is concerned that the growth of the fibroids may cause a miscarriage. Elizabeth is not cleared to exercise because of the incompetent cervix.

Elizabeth weighs 180 lb and is 61.5 inches tall. Her prepregnancy weight was 173 lb; her BMI is 32.0, and her blood pressure is 120/64 mm Hg. Her laboratory values are Hgb, 9.5 mg/dL; Hct, 30.3%; A1C, 5.8%; GCT, 154 mg/dL; OGTT: fasting, 89 mg/dL; 1 hour, 162 mg/dL; 2 hour, 153 mg/dL; 3 hour, 129 mg/dL. The maternal alpha-fetoprotein screen was negative.

Elizabeth's medications include a prenatal vitamin-mineral supplement, an iron supplement, and occasionally Tylenol when she experiences pain due to the fibroids.

Assessment

Elizabeth completes the nutrition assessment forms as requested by the RD. Her 24-hour recall is as follows:

- Breakfast (9:00 am): 1 small bowl of porridge made with 6 ounces milk
- Lunch (1:00 pm): 2 slices chicken breast with spinach and 1 cup rice
- Dinner (6:30 pm): 1 cup rice and peas with 3 pieces stewed beef and cabbage
- Snack (10:00 pm): 1 slice of cake

Elizabeth's estimated energy intake is 1,635 kcal/day, and her estimated energy requirement is 1,845 kcal/day.

Elizabeth was admitted to the hospital for incompetent cervix and cerclage. Her target blood glucose goals were < 95 mg/dL fasting and < 130 mg/dL 1 hour postprandial. She is instructed to self-monitor her blood glucose levels four times daily. Elizabeth states that she is unable to purchase a glucose meter or supplies because of her financial situation.

Intervention

The social worker refers Elizabeth to a diabetes foundation for a blood glucose meter and supplies. In the interim, Elizabeth will come to the health clinic four times a week for FBG and 2-hour postbreakfast blood glucose monitoring.

Elizabeth is instructed on an 1,845-kcal/day food plan, with emphasis on portion control and carbohydrate counting, using *First Step in Meal Planning*. The RD explains the effect of excessive carbohydrate intake on blood glucose levels. Elizabeth is encouraged to increase water intake. She is referred to the WIC and Food Stamp programs. Elizabeth will do the following:

- Keep food records
- Strive for weight-gain goals of $^2/_3$ lb/wk
- Use sugar substitute for regular sugar
- Strive for consistency with meals and snack times
- Include protein source for breakfast

Visit 2

Assessment

Elizabeth is at 17 weeks' gestation and weighs 181 lb. Her blood pressure is 143/78 mm Hg. She is concerned with cerclage and possible preterm delivery. She did not keep food records because she is now on bed rest. Her husband is now cooking, because of her limited activity. Her meals now consist primarily of starches and meat, with few vegetables. She is eating less, because most of the food is now fried. She finds it difficult to count carbohydrates with her husband's cooking methods.

The social worker is able to obtain a blood glucose monitor and supplies for 1 month. She will contact the insurance company to cover the costs of blood glucose monitoring, because of Elizabeth's medical condition.

Elizabeth's blood glucose ranges are 67–84 mg/dL fasting and 85–119 mg/dL 1 hour postprandial. Her random blood glucose level is 102 mg/dL.

Intervention

The RD reviews the food and blood glucose records and carbohydrate counting. Simple, quick, nutritious, and inexpensive recipes are downloaded from the Internet for Elizabeth to give to her husband. Elizabeth will do the following:

- Keep food records
- Be consistent with meal and snack times
- Resume carbohydrate counting

Visit 3

Assessment

Elizabeth is at 32 weeks' gestation. Her weight is 190 lb and her blood pressure is 121/71 mm Hg. Elizabeth was admitted to the hospital for the last 3 months, because of preterm labor and threatened abortion because of the fibroids. She continued the food plan during her hospital admission. She was discharged 1 week before Visit 3 (ie, at 31 weeks' gestation), with instructions to limit activity. She is happy because she is able to cook one meal a day and now eats leftovers for lunch. She is keeping food records and, as instructed by her obstetrician, has increased water intake to help prevent preterm labor. She has decreased blood glucose testing frequency, as instructed by her physician, because levels have been within normal limits.

Elizabeth has spoken by telephone with a WIC lactation consultant about breastfeeding. Her blood glucose ranges are 72–94 mg/dL fasting and 85–117 mg/dL 1 hour postprandial. The A1C value is 5.2%.

Intervention

The RD reviews Elizabeth's food and blood glucose records. She is instructed to use the simple recipes that the RD gave her at the last visit. Because these dishes are easy to prepare, Elizabeth will not have to overexert herself to have healthful meals. The RD also discusses with Elizabeth a weight-loss program to follow after delivery, to decrease risk of developing type 2 diabetes.

Visit 4

Assessment

Elizabeth is now at 35 weeks' gestation. She weighs 192 lb and her blood pressure is 114/76 mm Hg. Her blood glucose levels are within the normal range, and she is monitoring three times a week. Her random blood glucose value is 102 mg/dL.

Elizabeth is happy that, according to the last ultrasound, the baby has good interval growth and that the amniotic fluid level and biophysical profiles, which are performed twice weekly, are normal. She is following the food plan and has developed quick and simple recipes and will continue this after delivery.

Intervention

After reviewing Elizabeth's food and blood glucose records, no changes are made in her plan. Elizabeth will continue her present plan until delivery.

LACTO-VEGETARIAN PATIENT WITH PRETERM LABOR

Visit 1

Patient Data

Preema is a 29-year-old Indian woman who is referred to the RD for abnormal OGTT. She is at 28 weeks' gestation. Preema is gravida 4, para 2. She has an obstetric history of a spontaneous abortion at 5 weeks' gestation, 3 years ago. Her two previous deliveries were (a) 7 years ago, 37 weeks' gestation, 5-lb 9-oz boy, GDM A1 (diet controlled); and (b) 5 years ago, 36 weeks' gestation, 5-lb 11-oz girl, preterm labor 26–36 weeks, GDM A2 (diet and insulin controlled).

Preema is a lacto-vegetarian because of religion. She has a family history of diabetes (mother and paternal grandmother). She experienced nausea and vomiting during first trimester and was admitted for dehydration and given antiemetics, which were discontinued at 12 weeks.

Preema lives with her husband, two children, and parents. She works as a laboratory technician. Her husband is completing his cardiology fellowship. Her mother helps with after-school care. Preema does not smoke or drink and plans to breastfeed. She is not medically cleared to exercise because of her obstetrical history (two preterm deliveries).

Her medications include a prenatal vitamin-mineral supplement, an iron supplement, a calcium supplement (500 mg), and an antihistamine for allergies.

Preema weighs 138 lb and is 5 feet, 4 inches tall. Her prepregnancy weight is 120 lb, BMI is 20.6, and blood pressure is 120/64 mm Hg. Her laboratory values are Hgb, 11.3 mg/dL; Hct, 34.7%; GCT, 198 mg/dL; OGTT: fasting, 102 mg/dL; 1 hour, 193 mg/dL; 2 hour, 154 mg/dL; 3 hour, 129 mg/dL.

Assessment

Preema completes the initial nutrition assessment forms as directed by the RD. Her 24-hour recall is:

- Breakfast (8:30 am): $1/2$ bowl of cereal, 1 glass milk, $1/2$ cup tea with $1/2$ teaspoon sugar
- Snack (11:00 am): 6 pieces cantaloupe
- Lunch (1:00 pm): $1/2$ cup yogurt, 8 pieces pakoda, $1/2$ bowl yellow rice
- Snack (3:00 pm): $1/2$ bowl noodles made with chickpea flour, tea
- Dinner (6:30 pm): 4 rotis, $1/2$ bowl vegetables, $1/2$ bowl rice and dhal
- Snack (10:00 pm): 1 glass of milk

Her estimated energy requirement is 2,265 kcal, and her target blood glucose goals are <95 mg/dL fasting and <120 mg/dL 1 hour postprandial. She will self-monitor blood glucose four times daily (fasting and 1 hour postmeals).

Intervention

The RD instructs Preema on a 2,265-kcal food plan, consisting of three meals and three snacks. Instructions are provided on carbohydrate counting. The RD increases the protein intake to 20% of energy.

Preema will do the following:

- Keep food records
- Strive for a weight-gain goal of 1 lb/week
- Use sugar substitute to replace regular sugar

Visit 2

Assessment

Preema is at 30 weeks' gestation and weighs 138 lb. Her blood pressure is 112/66 mm Hg. She is concerned about possibly needing to self-inject insulin and has been consuming fewer calories than recommended. She complains of hunger after each meal. Food records show a daily average intake of 1,700 kcal. She consumes three meals and two snacks but eats only vegetables for lunch and does not eat a night snack. Her blood glucose levels are 75–94 mg/dL fasting and 78–115 mg/dL 1 hour postprandial.

Intervention

The RD reviews the food and blood glucose records. Three days of menus are developed to increase calorie intake to promote adequate weight gain. Weight-gain recommendations for the third trimester are also reviewed. Preema will do the following:

- Continue keeping food records
- Continue developing menus that will incorporate nutrition menus
- Resume carbohydrate counting

Visit 3

Assessment

Preema is at 32 weeks' gestation and her weight is 140 lb. Her blood pressure is 108/68 mm Hg. She was admitted to the hospital for preterm labor. She was started on terbutaline, a tocolytic agent that increased her blood glucose levels. She is now on an insulin plan of 6 units of regular insulin before dinner and 6 units of NPH before bedtime. She is carbohydrate counting and has developed a month's worth of menus and plans to rotate this schedule until delivery. Initially, she was afraid of injecting herself with insulin, but she recognizes the importance of optimal glycemic control. For example, when she ate ice cream for dessert at dinner, her blood glucose reading went to 168 mg/dL. Her blood glucose levels are 101–117 mg/dL fasting and 93–168 mg/dL 1 hour postprandial.

Intervention

The RD reviews the food records and blood glucose logs and reinforces the positive changes in Preema's eating habits. Instructions are given using *Exchange Lists for Meal Planning* and on incorporating other carbohydrates into the meal plan. The dinner and bedtime insulin doses were increased by her obstetrician. Preema will do the following:

- Use the *Exchange Lists* booklet to increase variety in her eating habits
- Continue to keep food records

Visit 4

Assessment

Preema is at 34 weeks' gestation. She weighs 142 lb, and her blood pressure is 98/65 mm Hg. Her blood glucose levels are 88–94 mg/dL fasting and 93–118 mg/dL 1 hour postprandial.

Preema is keeping her food records on a spreadsheet. She is using the *Exchange Lists* booklet to incorporate other carbohydrates into her food plan without changing the meal composition.

Intervention

No changes are made to the meal planning, and the RD emphasizes adequate fluid intake. Preema wants to continue receiving MNT by telephone and e-mail. She will e-mail her food records and blood glucose results to the RD once a week.

Postpartum

Assessment

Preema has returned for a postpartum visit because she is concerned about developing type 2 diabetes in the future, due to her family history. She delivered a 3,530-g boy at 39 weeks' gestation via cesarean section. Her insulin plan was discontinued before discharge because her blood glucose level was normal. Her weight is 132 lb, and her blood pressure is 108/68 mm Hg. Preema is following a modification of the same diet that she had during the pregnancy because she is breastfeeding.

Preema's 75-g OGTT at 6 weeks' postpartum is normal, and her fasting blood glucose was 91 mg/dL and her 2-hour postprandial value was 109 mg/dL.

Intervention

Preema is shown how to change her eating habits as the baby grows older and as she decreases the frequency of breastfeeding. Preema will follow-up with the RD once a month until she returns to her prepregnancy weight. She will also continue to check her blood glucose levels once a week at different times.

US-BORN MEXICAN AMERICAN CLIENT

Visit 1

Client Data

Yadira is a 32-year-old Mexican American woman referred for GDM. She is at 32 weeks' gestation and is gravida 2, para 1.

She works full-time at a desk job, and her activity level is very sedentary. She has a 3½-year-old daughter who was delivered by induction, because of Yadira's high blood glucose level. Yadira does not take prenatal supplements, although she will occasionally take her sister's vitamins and mineral supplements. She prefers American and Mexican foods.

Yadira weighs 198 lb at her first visit to the RD. Her reported prepregnancy weight was 143 lb. She is 5 feet, 8 inches tall, with a BMI of 21.29. Yadira reported that she was in an exercise and diet plan before and during pregnancy and had lost 12 pounds before discovering she was pregnant at 13 weeks' gestation. She stopped dieting and exercising and started to gain weight. She claims this gain is not due to overeating. Yadira is not monitoring her blood glucose levels.

Assessment

The 24-hour recall reveals inadequate intakes of vitamins A and C, secondary to inadequate intake of fruits and vegetables. Yadira eats at her mother's home four times per week and reports good-quality and healthful homemade food. A Mexican meal plan is discussed.

Intervention

Yadira is instructed on a 1,800-kcal/day plan, with 40% carbohydrate. A moderate fat intake is recommended because her actual fat intake ranges from 70 to 80 g, depending on whether she eats out or at her mother's home. The RD recommends fat intake of 50 g/day. Yadira is instructed on carbohydrate distribution per day, using a daily total of 180 g. To improve intakes of inadequate nutrients, the food plan includes an increase in fiber (corn tortillas instead of flour), fruits (two or three per day), and vegetables (up to five per day). Yadira is instructed to use nonfat milk (3 servings per day) to help reduce fat intake. She is instructed on blood glucose monitoring by the diabetes educator. Physical activity is discussed, and she is encouraged to walk, according to her physician's advice. Yadira is cooperative and demonstrates good understanding of the meal plan. The interview is conducted in English, as this was her preference.

The plans for follow-up include an evaluation of her SMBG, food record, and her sister's vitamin and mineral supplements. Yadira is a late entry for prenatal care and is knowledgeable about high blood glucose levels from her previous pregnancy with GDM. The RD instructs Yadira to bring her fasting and 1-hour postprandial blood glucose values to her next visit.

The dietitian lost contact with this client.

CLIENT WITH BMI OF 30 AND FAMILY HISTORY OF TYPE 2 DIABETES

First Visit

Client Data

Olga is a 35-year-old Spanish-speaking woman from Guatemala. She has a family history of type 2 diabetes (mother). She was referred to the RD at 20 weeks' gestation.

Olga's present weight is 209 lb. She is 5 feet, 5 inches tall, and her prepregnancy weight was 185 to 187 lb. Her BMI is 30. She smokes 3 to 4 cigarettes per day.

Assessment

Olga's initial 24-hour recall reveals very irregular eating habits. Her 24-hour recall was as follows:

- Morning (no specific time provided): 6 to 8 corn tortillas, 2 or 3 tablespoons of butter, coffee with milk and sugar
- Noon (no specific time provided): 1 Big Mac, 1 large regular Coke, 1 large order of french fries

Olga explains that the numbers she provided are approximations. She does not count the number of tortillas eaten nor does she measure amounts of food. Olga also explains that she does not eat dinner and has some snacks like bread and butter or a fruit or juice instead.

Olga has a 10-year-old daughter who is also obese. Both mother and daughter frequently eat at fast-food restaurants.

Intervention

The RD advises Olga on a 2,000-kcal/day diet. The carbohydrates are distributed among three meals and three snacks, with a total distribution of 40% of total energy intake. The RD explains the importance of regular meals and carbohydrate distribution. Olga needs to decrease her total fat from actual intake of about 100 g/day to 65 g/day.

Olga is introduced to home blood glucose monitoring. Olga will test her blood glucose four times daily: fasting and 1 hour postprandial. She appears to be cooperative. Her goals are as follows:

- Monitor her food records and blood glucose levels
- Record her activity levels
- Take prenatal vitamins

Visit 2

Assessment

Olga weighs 204 lb at 22 weeks' gestation, which is a loss of 4 lb. Her current diet shows an intake of about 1,800 to 2,000 kcal/day, with good carbohydrate distribution. She is eating three meals per day and a bedtime snack. She has improved her food quality and has decreased the fat as advised. Her activity level has increased to walking 20 minutes after meals.

Her blood glucose values are 85–100 mg/dL fasting and 87 to 120–130 mg/dL 1 hour postprandial, both of which are in normal ranges.

Intervention

The RD advises Olga to increase her daily protein intake by 3 ounces and drink 2 cups of nonfat milk. She agrees with the plan. She smokes less on some days only and will continue the effort to stop. No further changes are recommended for now.

Olga's goals are as follows:

- Monitor her food records and blood glucose levels
- Continue her physical activity
- Take prenatal vitamins

Olga changes residences and is not followed further at the clinical site.

UNCOOPERATIVE CLIENT WITH MORBID OBESITY

Visit 1

Client Data

Sandra is a 40-year-old woman referred to a diabetes and pregnancy center at 28 weeks' gestation after her private MD diagnoses her with GDM. This is her first pregnancy. She reports that she has been obese since childhood, has followed numerous diets, and has used medications to suppress her appetite. Her lowest weight was 140 lb, 13 years ago. She has stopped all diets and medications before planning to have a baby. Family history of diabetes is unknown.

Assessment

During her first visit, Sandra refuses to report a 24-hour food recall. She is very uncooperative and requests that the health team tell her what to do and what to eat. Her food preferences include chocolate, puddings, and desserts. She asks many questions regarding artificial sweeteners so that she can alter her cooking methods in preparing desserts.

Intervention

Sandra is instructed on the use of the home glucose meter and is given instructions on a meal plan and carbohydrate distribution. The RD advises Sandra to eat small meals, 3 to 4 hours apart. Portion sizes are discussed for carbohydrate distribution. Food models are used, including pictures and plates.

Sandra is instructed to keep food records for a week and to record all that she eats and drinks. Sandra is told of the importance to keep this record, which would be evaluated at the following appointment. She is advised to increase her activity level with 10- to 20-minute walks after meals if possible.

Visit 2

Assessment

Sandra is crying and upset because of difficulty with meal and blood glucose monitoring plans. She reports problems with the meter and difficulties in obtaining test strips because her insurance company would not pay for the strips. The meter is checked and is found to be working properly. Sandra expresses distress about being deprived of foods that she likes to eat. She is frustrated that she cannot eat her favorite desserts. She tells the RD that she may refuse to use insulin later in the pregnancy. Sandra did increase her activity, walking 15 to 20 minutes two times per day. She has a support belt to assist her with her stomach support for walks. Sandra's weight is stable, with a total gain of 10 lb.

Intervention

The RD evaluates Sandra's food record and finds that small frequent meals are the primary challenge with the GDM meal plan. The RD finds that Sandra kept the food record for the entire week and that there was good meal distribution and control in carbohydrate distribution. Sandra's blood glucose level was within normal ranges.

Because Sandra is using the food records as a way to comply with the instructions, the RD advises her to keep food records for 4 more weeks. She may not need to monitor blood glucose four times per day but only two, choosing the difficult meals. This plan is acceptable to her. However, she remains uncooperative, even with the support of the entire health care team and her husband. Sandra eventually delivers a boy weighing 3,910 g.

REFERENCES

1. American Dietetic Association. *Medical Nutrition Therapy Evidence-Based Guides for Practice: Nutrition Practice Guidelines for Gestational Diabetes Mellitus* [CD-ROM]. Chicago, Ill: American Dietetic Association; 2001.

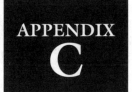

Energy, Carbohydrate, Protein, and Fat Content of Selected Foods

Food	Quantity	Grams/ Serving	Energy, kcal	Carb, g	Pro, g	Fat, g
Bread						
Bagel, plain	1/4 large (4″ diameter)	28	78	15.1	3.0	0.5
Bread sticks, crisp	4 sticks (4″ × 1/2″)	20	82	13.7	2.4	1.9
Bread, pumpernickel, dark	1 slice	32	80	15.2	2.8	1.0
Bread, reduced-calorie white	2 slices	46	95	20.4	4.0	1.1
Bread, rye, light or dark	1 slice	32	83	15.5	2.7	1.1
Bread, white	1 slice	25	67	12.4	2.0	0.9
Bread, whole-wheat	1 slice	28	69	12.9	2.7	1.2
Bun or roll, hamburger	1/2 small bun	22	62	10.8	1.8	1.1
English muffin	1/2 muffin	28	67	13.1	2.2	0.5
Pancake plain, frozen, reheated	1 pancake (4″ diameter)	36	82	15.7	1.9	1.2
Pita bread, white	1/2 pita	30	82	16.7	2.7	0.4
Roll, plain dinner	1 roll	28	85	14.3	2.4	2.1
Tortilla, corn	1 medium (6″ diameter)	24	53	11.2	1.4	0.6
Tortilla, flour, 6″ diameter	1 tortilla	30	98	16.7	2.6	2.1
Cereals and Grains						
All-bran cereal	1/2 cup	31	81	22.9	3.9	1.0
Bulgur wheat, cooked	1/2 cup	91	76	16.9	2.8	0.2
Corn flakes	3/4 cup	21	76	18.1	1.5	0.2
Couscous, prepared	1/3 cup	52	58	12.1	2.0	0.1
Cream of rice, cooked	1/2 cup	122	63	13.9	1.1	0.1
Cream of wheat, cooked	1/2 cup	126	67	13.9	1.9	0.3
Granola cereal, low-fat	1/4 cup	22	86	18.0	1.8	1.1
Grape-nuts cereal	1/4 cup	29	104	23.6	3.1	0.6
Grits, cooked	1/2 cup	121	73	15.7	1.7	0.2
Kasha (buckwheat groats), roasted, cooked	1/2 cup	84	77	16.7	2.8	0.5
Macaroni, cooked firm	1/3 cup	46	65	13.1	2.2	0.3
Muesli	1/4 cup	21	74	15.1	1.9	1.1
Oatmeal, cooked	1/2 cup	117	73	12.6	3.0	1.2
Pasta, cooked	1/3 cup	43	62	12.8	2.1	0.3
Puffed rice cereal	1 1/2 cups	21	80	18.4	1.5	0.2
Puffed wheat cereal	1 1/2 cups	18	66	13.8	2.9	0.4
Rice, brown, cooked	1/3 cup	64	71	14.8	1.7	0.6
Rice, white, long-grain, cooked	1/3 cup	52	68	14.7	1.4	0.1
Shredded wheat	1/2 cup	24	83	20.3	2.5	0.3
Spaghetti, cooked firm	1/3	46	65	13.1	2.2	0.3
Wheat germ, toasted	3 Tbsp	21	80	10.4	6.1	2.2
Starchy vegetables						
Beans, baked	1/3 cup	84	78	17.2	4.0	0.4
Corn on cob, cooked	1/2 large ear	72	66	16.0	2.2	0.5
Corn, canned, drained	1/2 cup	82	66	15.2	2.1	0.8
Corn, frozen, cooked	1/2 cup	82	66	16.0	2.3	0.4
Peas, green, frozen, cooked	1/2 cup	80	62	11.4	4.1	0.2
Plantain, ripe, cooked	1/2 cup, slices	77	89	24.0	0.6	0.1
Potato, baked with skin	3 oz	85	79	18.0	2.1	0.1
Potato, fresh, mashed, made with milk	1/2 cup	105	85	18.7	2.0	0.4
Potato, white, peeled, cooked	3 oz	85	73	17.0	1.5	0.1
Squash, winter, cooked	1 cup, cubes	205	80	17.9	1.8	1.3
Yams, cooked	1/2 cup, cubes	68	79	18.8	1.0	0.1

Food	Quantity	Grams/ Serving	Energy, kcal	Carb, g	Pro, g	Fat, g
Crackers and snacks						
Crackers, animal	8 crackers	20	89	14.8	1.4	2.8
Crackers, graham	3 crackers	21	89	16.1	1.4	2.1
Crackers, oyster	20 crackers	20	87	14.3	1.8	2.4
Crackers, saltine	6 crackers	18	78	12.9	1.7	2.1
Crackers, whole-wheat, reduced-fat	5 triscuits	20	80	15.0	1.8	2.0
Matzoh	3/4 oz	21	83	17.6	2.1	0.3
Melba toast	4 pieces	20	78	15.3	2.4	0.6
Popcorn, popped, no salt/fat added	3 cups	24	92	18.7	2.9	1.0
Potato chips, baked	3/4 oz	21	82	17.2	1.5	1.1
Potato chips, nonfat	3/4 oz	21	56	13.5	1.5	0.0
Pretzels, sticks/rings	3/4 oz	21	80	16.6	1.9	0.7
Rice cakes	2 cakes	18	70	14.7	1.5	0.5
Tortilla chips, baked (low-fat)	3/4 oz	21	83	18.0	2.3	0.7
Beans, peas, and lentils						
Beans, garbanzo (chickpeas), cooked	1/2 cup	82	134	22.5	7.3	2.1
Beans, kidney, canned	1/2 cup	128	104	19.0	6.7	0.4
Beans, pinto, cooked	1/2 cup	85	116	21.8	7.0	0.4
Beans, white, cooked	1/2 cup	90	125	22.6	8.8	0.3
Lentils, cooked	1/2 cup	99	115	19.9	8.9	0.4
Miso paste	3 Tbsp	52	107	14.5	6.1	3.2
Peas, black-eyed, cooked	1/2 cup	86	100	17.9	6.6	0.5
Peas, split, cooked	1/2 cup	98	116	20.7	8.2	0.4
Starchy foods prepared with fat						
Biscuit, baked, 2 1/2" diameter	1 biscuit	35	127	17.0	2.2	5.8
Cornbread, baked	1 cube (2")	57	152	24.8	3.8	4.0
Crackers, round butter type	6 crackers	18	90	11.0	1.3	4.6
Croutons	1 cup	30	122	22.1	3.6	2.0
Granola	1/4 cup	28	125	19.0	2.1	4.9
Hummus	1/3 cup	83	137	11.8	6.5	7.9
Popcorn, microwave	3	18	111	9.6	1.6	7.2
Potato chips	3/4 oz	21	114	11.2	1.5	7.3
Potatoes, french-fried, frozen, oven-baked	1 cup	57	114	17.8	1.8	4.3
Sandwich crackers, peanut butter	3 sandwiches	21	102	12.3	2.3	5.0
Stuffing, bread, prepared	1/3 cup	66	117	14.3	2.1	5.7
Taco shells	2 shells	27	124	16.6	1.9	6.0
Tortilla chips	3/4 oz	21	106	13.4	1.5	5.6
Fruit						
Apple, unpeeled	1 apple	106	63	16.2	0.2	0.4
Applesauce, unsweetened	1/2 cup	122	52	13.8	0.2	0.1
Apricots, dried	8 halves	28	67	17.3	1.0	0.1
Apricots, fresh	4 apricots	140	67	15.6	2.0	0.5
Banana, fresh, small	1 banana	72	66	16.9	0.7	0.3
Blackberries, fresh	3/4 cup	108	56	13.8	0.8	0.4
Blueberries, fresh	3/4 cup	109	61	15.4	0.7	0.4
Cantaloupe, fresh	1 cup	160	56	13.4	1.4	0.4
Cherries, sweet, fresh	12 cherries	82	59	13.7	1.0	0.8
Dates	3 dates	25	69	18.5	0.5	0.1
Figs, dried	1 1/2 oz figs	28	71	18.2	0.9	0.3

Food	Quantity	Grams/ Serving	Energy, kcal	Carb, g	Pro, g	Fat, g
Figs, fresh, medium	2 figs	100	74	19.2	0.8	0.3
Fruit cocktail, canned, juice pack	1/2 cup	124	60	14.0	0.0	0.0
Grapefruit, fresh	1/2 grapefruit	166	53	13.4	1.0	0.2
Grapes, fresh seedless, small	17 grapes	85	60	15.1	0.6	0.5
Honeydew melon, fresh	1 cup	170	60	15.6	0.8	0.2
Kiwi	1 large	91	56	13.5	0.9	0.4
Mandarin oranges, canned, juice pack	3/4 cup	187	69	17.9	1.2	0.1
Mango, fresh, small	1/2 mango	104	68	17.7	0.5	0.3
Nectarine, fresh, small	1 nectarine	136	67	16.0	1.3	0.6
Orange, fresh	1 orange	131	62	15.4	1.2	0.2
Papaya, fresh	1 cup	140	55	13.7	0.9	0.2
Peach, fresh	1 peach	147	63	16.3	1.0	0.1
Pear, fresh	1/2 pear	105	62	15.9	0.4	0.4
Pineapple, canned, juice pack	1/2 cup	124	74	19.5	0.5	0.1
Pineapple, fresh	3/4 cup	116	57	14.4	0.5	0.5
Plum, fresh	2 plums	132	73	17.2	1.0	0.8
Plums, dried (prunes)	3 prunes	25	60	15.6	0.7	0.1
Raisins, dark, seedless	2 Tbsp	18	54	14.2	0.6	0.1
Raspberries, fresh	1 cup	123	60	14.2	1.1	0.7
Strawberries, fresh	1 1/4 cups	190	57	13.3	1.2	0.7
Tangerine, fresh	2 tangerines	168	74	18.8	1.1	0.3
Watermelon, fresh	1 1/4 cups	190	61	13.6	1.2	0.8
Fruit juice, unsweetened						
Apple juice or cider, canned/bottle	1/2 cup	124	58	14.5	0.1	0.1
Cranberry juice cocktail	1/3 cup	83	48	12.0	0.0	0.1
Cranberry juice cocktail, reduced-calorie (light)	1 cup	237	40	10.0	0.0	0.0
Fruit juice blends, 100% juice	1/3 cup	83	50	11.6	0.0	0.1
Grape juice	1/3 cup	83	50	12.5	0.5	0.1
Grapefruit juice, canned	1/2 cup	124	47	11.1	0.6	0.1
Orange juice, fresh	1/2 cup	124	56	12.9	0.9	0.2
Pineapple juice, canned	1/2 cup	125	70	17.2	0.4	0.1
Prune juice, bottled	1/3 cup	84	59	14.7	0.5	0.0
Nonfat and low-fat milk						
Buttermilk, low-fat	1 cup	245	99	11.7	8.1	2.2
Milk, low-fat	1 cup	244	102	11.7	8.0	2.6
Milk, evaporated nonfat	1/2 cup	128	100	14.5	9.7	0.3
Milk, nonfat	1 cup	245	86	11.9	8.4	0.4
Milk, nonfat dry	1/3 cup	22	80	11.7	7.9	0.2
Soy milk, low-fat/nonfat	1 cup	245	87	14.6	3.7	1.2
Yogurt, light nonfat, sweetener and fructose	6 oz (2/3 cup)	170	92	17.0	6.0	0.0
Yogurt, nonfat, plain	6 oz (2/3 cup)	170	90	14.0	9.0	0.0
Reduced-fat milk						
Milk, reduced-fat	1 cup	244	121	11.7	8.1	4.7
Yogurt, low-fat, plain	6 oz (2/3 cup)	170	110	14.0	9.0	2.5
Whole milk						
Milk, evaporated, whole	1/2 cup	126	169	12.6	8.6	9.5

Food	Quantity	Grams/ Serving	Energy, kcal	Carb, g	Pro, g	Fat, g
Milk, goat, whole	1 cup	244	168	10.9	8.7	10.1
Milk, whole	1 cup	244	150	11.4	8.0	8.1
Sweets, desserts, and other carbohydrates						
Angel food cake, unfrosted	1 slice	53	142	31.5	4.0	0.1
Brownie, small, unfrosted	1 brownie	28	115	18.1	1.4	4.6
Cake, frosted	1 square (2″)	50	175	29.2	1.6	6.4
Cake, unfrosted	1 square (2″)	32	97	16.6	1.5	3.1
Cookies, sandwich, cream filling	2 cookies	20	94	14.1	1.0	4.2
Cookies, small	2 cookies	24	114	15.2	1.4	5.6
Cranberry sauce, canned, sugar added	1/4 cup	69	104	26.8	0.1	0.1
Cupcake, frosted, small	1 cupcake	48	172	28.4	2.2	6.0
Doughnut, cake-type, plain, medium	1 doughnut	47	198	23.4	2.3	10.8
Fruit juice bar, frozen, 100% juice	1 bar	92	75	18.6	1.1	0.1
Fruit snacks/rolls, chewy	1 roll	21	78	17.7	0.2	1.5
Fruit spread (100% fruit)	1 1/2 Tbsp	28	60	15.0	0.2	0.0
Gelatin, regular, prepared	1/2 cup	135	80	18.9	1.6	0.0
Gingersnap cookies, regular	3 cookies	21	87	16.1	1.2	2.1
Granola bar	1 bar	28	134	18.3	2.9	5.6
Honey	1 Tbsp	21	64	17.3	0.1	0.0
Ice cream	1/2 cup	66	133	15.6	2.3	7.3
Jam or preserves, regular	1 Tbsp	20	48	12.9	0.1	0.0
Milk, chocolate, whole	1 cup	250	208	25.9	7.9	8.5
Pasta sauce	1/2 cup	128	110	17.0	2.0	4.0
Pie, fruit, 2 crust	1 slice (1/6 pie)	117	284	42.4	2.2	12.5
Pie, pumpkin or custard	1 slice (1/8 pie)	80	168	19.3	3.8	8.4
Pudding, regular (reduced-fat milk)	1/2 cup	140	144	26.5	4.3	2.6
Rice milk, nonfat or reduced-fat, plain	1 cup	252	90	18.0	1.1	1.5
Salad dressing, nonfat, large serving	1/4 cup	64	80	18.0	0.1	0.0
Sherbet	1/2 cup	96	132	29.2	1.1	1.9
Sorbet	1/2 cup	96	136	32.3	0.4	0.0
Spaghetti sauce	1/2 cup	125	136	20.0	2.0	6.0
Sugar, white, granulated	1 Tbsp	12	46	12.0	0.0	0.0
Sweet roll	1 roll	71	264	36.1	4.4	11.6
Syrup, reduced-caloric/light	2 Tbsp	33	40	10.0	0.0	0.0
Syrup, regular, large serving	1/4 cup	60	200	53.0	0.0	0.0
Syrup, regular, small serving	1 Tbsp	20	50	13.2	0.0	0.0
Yogurt, frozen, nonfat	1/3 cup	44	59	12.5	2.0	0.0
Yogurt, frozen, vanilla	1/2 cup	65	100	17.0	2.6	2.5
Yogurt, low-fat, with fruit	1 cup	248	253	47.2	10.0	2.8
Nonstarchy vegetables						
Artichoke, cooked	1/2 artichoke	60	30	7.3	2.5	0.4
Asparagus, frozen, cooked	1/2 cup	90	25	4.4	2.7	0.4
Bean sprouts, raw	1 cup	100	30	5.9	3.0	0.2
Beans, canned, drained (green, wax)	1/2 cup	68	14	3.1	0.8	0.1
Beets, canned, drained	1/2 cup	85	26	6.1	0.8	0.1
Broccoli, fresh, cooked	1/2 cup	78	22	4.0	2.3	0.3
Cabbage, fresh, cooked	1/2 cup	75	17	3.3	0.8	0.3
Carrots, raw	1 cup	122	52	12.4	1.3	0.2
Cauliflower, fresh, raw	1 cup	100	25	5.2	2.0	0.2
Celery, fresh, raw	1 cup	124	20	4.5	0.9	0.2

Food	Quantity	Grams/ Serving	Energy, kcal	Carb, g	Pro, g	Fat, g
Collard greens, fresh, cooked	½ cup	95	26	5.8	1.3	0.2
Cucumber	1 cup	104	14	2.9	0.7	0.1
Eggplant, fresh, cooked	½ cup	48	13	3.2	0.4	0.1
Kale, fresh, cooked	½ cup	65	21	3.7	1.2	0.3
Mixed vegetables (no corn, peas, pasta	½ cup	54	20	3.3	1.0	0.1
Onions, fresh, cooked	½ cup	105	46	10.7	1.4	0.2
Pea pods (snow peas), fresh, cooked	½ cup	80	34	5.6	2.6	0.2
Pepper, green, raw, sliced	1 cup	92	25	5.9	0.8	0.2
Spinach, fresh, raw	1 cup	30	7	1.0	0.9	0.1
Squash, summer, fresh, cooked	½ cup	90	18	3.9	0.8	0.3
Tomato juice	½ cup	122	21	5.2	0.9	0.1
Tomato sauce	½ cup	122	37	8.8	1.6	0.2
Tomato, raw	1 cup	180	38	8.4	1.5	0.6
Turnip greens, fresh, cooked	½ cup	72	14	3.1	0.8	0.2
Vegetable juice	½ cup	121	25	5.5	0.8	0.1
Zucchini squash, fresh, cooked	½ cup	90	14	3.5	0.6	0.0
Very lean meat and substitutes						
Cheese, cheddar, nonfat	1 oz	30	45	2.0	9.0	0.0
Chicken breast, roasted, no skin	1 oz	28	47	0.0	8.8	1.0
Cod fillet, cooked	1 oz	28	30	0.0	6.5	0.2
Cornish game hen, whole bird, cooked, no skin	1 oz	28	38	0.0	6.6	1.1
Cottage cheese, nonfat	¼ cup	56	40	2.5	7.0	0.0
Egg substitute	¼ cup	61	30	1.0	6.0	0.0
Egg white	2 egg whites	67	34	0.7	7.0	0.0
Flounder, cooked	1 oz	28	33	0.0	6.8	0.4
Hot dog, less than 1 g fat/oz	1 oz	28	30	2.5	3.5	0.8
Kidney, beef, simmered	1 oz	28	41	0.3	7.2	1.0
Sausage, smoked, low-fat (turkey, pork, beef)	1 oz	28	40	3.0	3.5	1.3
Scallops, fresh, steamed	1 oz	28	30	0.7	4.6	0.9
Shrimp, fresh, cooked in water	1 oz	28	28	0.0	5.9	0.3
Tuna, canned in water, drained	1 oz	28	33	0.0	7.2	0.2
Turkey breast, roasted	1 oz	28	38	0.0	8.5	0.2
Turkey ham	1 oz	28	36	0.1	5.4	1.4
Lean meat and substitutes						
Beef tenderloin, lean, broiled	1 oz	28	60	0.0	8.0	2.8
Beef, flank steak, lean, cooked	1 oz	28	59	0.0	7.7	2.9
Beef, ground round, cooked	1 oz	28	56	0.0	10.2	1.4
Beef, round steak, lean, cooked	1 oz	28	59	0.0	8.9	2.3
Beef, sirloin, lean, cooked	1 oz	28	54	0.0	8.6	1.9
Cheese, cheddar, low-fat	1 oz	28	49	0.5	6.9	2.0
Chicken, dark meat, no skin, roasted	1 oz	28	58	0.0	7.7	2.8
Chicken, light meat with skin, roasted	1 oz	28	63	0.0	8.2	3.1
Cottage cheese, creamed, 4.5% milkfat	¼ cup	52	54	1.4	6.5	2.3
Duck, domestic, no skin, roasted	1 oz	28	57	0.0	6.6	3.2
Goose, no skin, roasted	1 oz	28	67	0.0	8.2	3.6
Ham, cured, roasted	1 oz	28	44	0.0	7.1	1.6
Ham, fresh, baked	1 oz	28	60	0.0	8.3	2.7
Hot dog or frankfurter, low-fat	1 frankfurter	50	70	6.0	6.4	2.5
Lamb loin, roast/chop, cooked	1 oz	28	61	0.0	8.5	2.8

Food	Quantity	Grams/ Serving	Energy, kcal	Carb, g	Pro, g	Fat, g
Liver, chicken, cooked	1 oz	28	44	0.2	6.9	1.5
Oysters, medium, cooked	6 oysters	42	58	3.3	5.9	2.1
Pork chop, cooked	1 oz	28	57	0.0	8.4	2.4
Pork tenderloin, cooked	1 oz	28	46	0.0	8.0	1.4
Salmon, canned, solids and liquids	1 oz	28	39	0.0	5.6	1.7
Salmon, fresh, broiled or baked	1 oz	28	61	0.0	7.7	3.1
Sardines, medium, packed in oil, drained	2 sardines	24	50	0.0	5.9	2.7
Tuna, canned in oil, drained	1 oz	28	53	0.0	7.5	2.3
Turkey, dark meat, no skin, cooked	1 oz	28	53	0.0	8.1	2.0
Veal loin, chop, cooked	1 oz	28	64	0.0	9.5	2.6
Medium-fat meat and substitutes						
Beef patty, ground, lean, pan broiled (80% lean)	1 oz	28	70	0.0	6.8	4.5
Beef patty, ground, regular, pan-broiled (75% lean)	1 oz	28	70	0.0	6.6	4.7
Beef, prime rib, roasted	1 oz	28	83	0.0	7.7	5.5
Beef, short ribs, cooked	1 oz	28	83	0.0	8.7	5.1
Cheese, mozzarella (part nonfat milk)	1 oz	28	72	0.8	6.9	4.5
Cheese, ricotta (part nonfat milk)	1/4 cup	62	85	3.2	7.0	4.9
Chicken, dark meat with skin, roasted	1 oz	28	72	0.0	7.3	4.5
Chicken, with skin, roasted	1 oz	28	68	0.0	7.7	3.8
Egg, fresh	1 egg	50	75	0.6	6.2	5.0
Lamb rib, roasted	1 oz	28	66	0.0	7.4	3.8
Meatloaf	1 oz	28	65	1.5	6.0	3.9
Pork cutlet, cooked	1 oz	28	71	0.0	7.9	4.2
Tempeh	1/4 cup	42	84	7.2	8.0	3.2
Tofu	4 oz	124	94	2.3	10.0	5.9
Turkey, ground, cooked	1 oz	28	67	0.0	7.7	3.7
Veal cutlet, lean, cooked	1 oz	28	57	0.0	10.4	1.4
High-fat meat and substitutes						
Bacon, fried, drained	3 slices	19	108	0.1	5.8	9.4
Bologna	1 oz	28	90	0.8	3.3	8.0
Cheese, American	1 oz	28	93	2.1	5.6	7.0
Cheese, cheddar-type	1 oz	28	114	0.4	7.1	9.4
Cheese, swiss, regular	1 oz	28	107	1.0	8.1	7.8
Hot dog	1 hot dog	45	144	1.1	5.1	13.1
Hot dog, turkey	1 hot dog	45	102	0.7	6.4	8.0
Peanut butter	1 Tbsp	16	95	3.1	4.0	8.2
Pork sausage, fresh, cooked	1 oz	28	104	0.3	5.6	8.8
Pork spareribs, cooked, lean and fat	1 oz	28	112	0.0	8.2	8.6
Salami	1 oz	28	71	0.6	4.0	5.7
Sausage, Italian, cooked	1 oz	28	91	0.4	5.7	7.3
Monounsaturated fats						
Almonds, dry roasted	6 almonds	8	47	1.9	1.3	4.1
Avocado	2 Tbsp	28	45	2.1	0.6	4.3
Cashews, salted	6 cashews	9	52	2.9	1.4	4.2
Oil, olive	1 tsp	4	40	0.0	0.0	4.5
Olives, large, ripe, pitted	8 olives	35	40	2.2	0.3	3.7
Peanut butter	1/2 Tbsp	8	49	1.6	2.1	4.2

Food	Quantity	Grams/ Serving	Energy, kcal	Carb, g	Pro, g	Fat, g
Peanuts, dry roasted, no salt	10 peanuts	10	59	2.2	2.4	5.0
Tahini	2 tsp	10	60	2.1	1.7	5.4
Polyunsaturated fats						
Margarine	1 tsp	5	34	0.0	0.0	3.8
Margarine, light, stick	1 Tbsp	14	48	0.1	0.1	5.4
Mayonnaise	1 tsp	5	33	0.1	0.1	3.7
Mayonnaise, light	1 Tbsp	15	50	1.0	0.1	5.0
Miracle Whip salad dressing	2 tsp	10	47	1.3	0.1	4.7
Oil, corn	1 tsp	4	40	0.0	0.0	4.5
Salad dressing, regular	1 Tbsp	15	64	1.9	0.5	6.1
Sunflower seeds, dry roasted	1 Tbsp	8	47	1.9	1.5	4.0
Saturated fats						
Bacon, fried, drained	1 slice	6	35	0.0	1.8	3.0
Butter	1 tsp	5	34	0.0	0.0	3.8
Butter, whipped	2 tsp	6	43	0.0	0.1	4.9
Chitterlings, boiled	2 Tbsp	14	42	0.0	1.4	4.0
Coconut milk	1 Tbsp	15	34	0.8	0.3	3.6
Cream cheese	1 Tbsp	14	51	0.4	1.1	5.1
Cream, half & half	2 Tbsp	30	39	1.3	0.9	3.5
Sour cream, regular	2 Tbsp	24	51	1.0	0.8	5.0
Nonfat or reduced-fat foods						
Cream cheese, nonfat	1 Tbsp	16	15	1.0	2.5	0.0
Creamer, nondairy, powder, regular	2 tsp	4	22	2.2	0.2	1.4
Margarine, nonfat	4 Tbsp	56	20	0.5	0.0	0.0
Margarine, reduced-fat	1 tsp	5	16	0.0	0.0	1.8
Mayonnaise, nonfat	1 Tbsp	14	10	2.0	0.2	0.0
Mayonnaise, reduced-fat	1 tsp	5	13	1.0	0.0	1.0
Miracle Whip nonfat salad dressing	1 Tbsp	16	15	3.0	0.0	0.0
Miracle Whip, reduced-fat	1 tsp	5	20	1.2	0.0	1.7
Salad dressing, nonfat	1 Tbsp	16	20	4.5	0.0	0.0
Salad dressing, Italian, nonfat	2 Tbsp	31	15	3.2	0.2	0.0
Sour cream, reduced-fat	1 Tbsp	16	18	2.0	0.5	1.0
Whipped topping, light	2 Tbsp	8	20	2.0	0.0	1.0
Whipped topping, regular	1 Tbsp	4	12	1.0	0.1	0.8
Sugar-free foods						
Gelatin dessert, sugar-free, prepared	1/4 cup	117	8	0.8	1.3	0.0
Gelatin, unflavored	1 envelope	7	23	0.0	6.0	0.0
Jelly/preserves, low- or reduced-sugar	2 tsp	11	16	4.0	0.0	0.0
Syrup, sugar-free	2 Tbsp	15	9	2.3	0.0	0.0
Drinks						
Cocoa, powder, unsweetened	1 Tbsp	5	12	2.9	1.1	0.8
Coffee, brewed	1 cup	236	5	1.1	0.1	0.0
Diet soft drinks, sugar-free	1 can	355	4	0.3	0.4	0.0
Tea, brewed	1 cup	237	3	0.5	0.0	0.0
Condiments						
Catsup (ketchup), tomato	1 Tbsp	15	16	4.1	0.2	0.1
Lemon juice	1 Tbsp	15	3	1.0	0.1	0.0

Food	Quantity	Grams/ Serving	Energy, kcal	Carb, g	Pro, g	Fat, g
Lime Juice	1 Tbsp	15	3	1.0	0.0	0.0
Mustard, prepared	1 tsp	5	3	0.4	0.2	0.2
Pickles, dill	1½ medium (3¾")	98	17	4.0	0.6	0.2
Relish, sweet pickle	1 Tbsp	15	20	5.3	0.1	0.1
Salsa	¼ cup	65	15	3.2	0.7	0.1
Soy sauce	1 Tbsp	18	7	1.4	0.4	0.0
Soy sauce, light	1 Tbsp	18	7	1.4	0.4	0.0
Taco sause	1 Tbsp	16	7	1.3	0.2	0.1
Vinegar	1 Tbsp	10	1	0.6	0.0	0.0
Yogurt, plain, nonfat milk, small serving	2 Tbsp	31	17	2.4	1.8	0.1
Combination foods						
Chili with beans	1 cup	253	256	21.9	24.6	8.3
Chow mein, no noodles or rice	2 cups	530	160	12.0	16.0	7.0
Lasagna with meat and sauce	1 cup	227	293	27.9	19.7	11.4
Macaroni and cheese	1 cup	253	283	35.4	10.8	11.0
Meatless burger, soy-based	1 patty	90	140	8.0	18.0	4.1
Pizza, cheese, thin crust, frozen	1¼ of 12"	126	291	33.0	13.5	12.5
Pot pie, double crust	1 pie (7 oz)	198	390	39.3	9.7	21.3
Soup, bean	1 cup	247	116	19.8	5.6	1.5
Soup, chicken noodle, made w/water	1 cup	241	75	9.4	4.0	2.5
Soup, cream of mushroom, made w/water	1 cup	244	129	9.3	2.3	9.0
Soup, split pea, made w/water	½ cup	127	95	14.0	5.2	2.2
Soup, tomato, made w/water	1 cup	244	85	16.6	2.0	1.9
Soup, vegetable beef, made w/water	1 cup	244	78	10.2	5.6	1.9
Fast foods						
Burrito	1 burrito, small	178	364	48.0	15.0	13.0
Chicken breast/wing, breaded and fried	1 chicken (¼)	163	494	19.6	35.7	29.5
Chicken nuggets, plain	6 nuggets	102	290	15.5	16.9	17.7
Chicken wings, hot	6 drummettes	144	443	0.3	37.5	31.3
Fish sandwich with tartar sauce	1 sandwich	158	431	41.0	16.9	22.8
French fries	1 serving (5 oz)	145	429	57.0	5.0	20.0
Grilled chicken sandwich	1 sandwich	182	285	35.0	25.0	5.0
Hamburger, large, with bun	1 hamburger	137	426	31.7	22.6	22.9
Hamburger, regular, with bun, plain	1 hamburger	90	275	30.5	12.3	11.8
Hot dog with bun, plain	1 hot dog	98	242	18.0	10.4	14.5
Pizza, individual pan	1 pizza	327	722	70.0	33.0	34.0
Pizza, meat, thin crust, fast food	1¼ of 12"	164	426	40.6	20.6	21.9
Soft-serve cone, regular	1 cone	142	226	33.2	5.4	8.4
Submarine sandwich	1 sub (6")	228	456	51.0	21.8	18.6
Taco, small, hard shell	1 taco (2¾ oz)	78	210	18.0	9.0	12.0
Taco, soft shell	1 taco (3 oz)	99	220	19.0	12.0	11.0

Abbreviations: Carb, carbohydrate; Pro, protein.
Source: Adapted from Wheeler ML. Nutrient database for 2003 exchange lists for meal planning. *J Am Diet Assoc.* 2003;103:894–920. Used with permission.

Glossary

acesulfame potassium. A dietary sweetener with no calories and no nutritional value. Also known as acesulfame-K.

agenesis. Absence or failure of formation or imperfect development of any body part.

alpha-fetoprotein. A fetal blood protein found in the amniotic fluid of pregnant women; very low levels tend to be associated with Down syndrome in the fetus, and very high levels tend to be associated with neural tube defects.

alpha-glucosidase inhibitors. Class of oral medications for type 2 diabetes that blocks enzymes that digest starches in food. The result is a slower and lower rise in blood glucose throughout the day, especially right after meals.

amniocentesis. Transabdominal aspiration of fluid from the amniotic sac.

anencephaly. Congenital absence of all or a major portion of the brain. This condition is incompatible with life.

antidiabetic agent. A substance that helps control blood glucose level in the body.

antiemetic. An agent used to prevent or control vomiting.

aspartame. A noncarbohydrate compound, $C_{14}H_{18}N_2O_5$, which is formed from the amino acids phenylalanine and aspartic acid and is used as a low-calorie sweetener.

aspart insulin. *See* rapid-acting insulin.

beta-sympathomimetics. A tocolytic agent used to relax uterine smooth muscles.

biguanides. A class of oral medications, used to treat type 2 diabetes, which lowers blood glucose by reducing the amount of glucose produced by the liver and by helping the body respond better to insulin.

biophysical profile. A test used to assess fetal heart rate, breathing pattern, body movements, muscle tone, and the amniotic fluid level. It combines a nonstress test with an ultrasound.

bolus. Additional amount of insulin taken to cover an expected rise in blood glucose, often related to a meal or a snack.

calcium channel blockers. Class of drugs that block the flow of calcium (either in nerve cell conduction or smooth muscle contraction) of the heart.

cannula. A small tube for insertion into a body cavity or into a duct or vessel.

cerclage. Any of several procedures for increasing tissue resistance in a functionally incompetent uterine cervical os, usually involving reinforcement with a nonabsorbable suture.

continuous subcutaneous insulin infusion (CSII). The constant, continuous infusion of a rapid-acting insulin, driven by mechanical force and delivered via a needle or soft cannula under the skin.

contraction stress test. A test to check the fetal heart rate when the mother has a uterine contraction.

creatine. A white crystalline nitrogenous substance, $C_4H9N_3O_2$, found especially in the muscles of vertebrates, either free or as phosphocreatine.

creatinine. A white crystalline, strongly basic compound, $C_4H_7N_3O$, formed from creatine and found especially in muscle, blood, and urine.

creatinine clearance. A test that compares the level of creatinine in urine with the creatinine level in the blood, usually based on assessments of a 24-hour urine sample and a blood sample drawn at the end of the 24-hour period.

cultural competence. A set of academic and interpersonal skills that allow individuals to increase their understanding and appreciation of cultural differences and similarities within, among, and between groups.

cultural sensitivity. An awareness of one's own cultural beliefs, assumptions, customs, and values, as well as those of other cultural groups.

dystocia. A slow or difficult labor or delivery.

eclampsia. Onset of convulsions or coma in a previously diagnosed preeclamptic patient.

euglycemia. See *normoglycemia*.

facilitated diffusion. A process by which carrier (transport) proteins in the cell membrane transport substances into or out of cells down a concentration gradient.

fundal height. The distance from the fundus to the pelvic bone.

fundus. The upper large end of the uterus.

gestational diabetes mellitus (GDM). Any degree of glucose intolerance, with onset or first recognition during pregnancy.

glargine insulin. See *very-long-acting insulin*.

glucose challenge test (GCT). A screening test usually performed between 24 and 28 weeks of pregnancy, to check for gestational diabetes.

gluconeogenesis. Formation of glucose within the animal body, especially by the liver, from substances (such as fats and protein) other than carbohydrates.

GLUT transporters. Glucose transporter molecules that transport glucose into cells via placental diffusion.

glyburide. An oral medication used to treat type 2 diabetes. It lowers blood glucose by helping the pancreas make more insulin and by helping the body better use the insulin it makes. Belongs to the class of medicines called sulfonylureas.

glycated serum protein. A test that measures the number of blood glucose molecules linked to protein molecules in the blood. The test provides information on the average blood glucose level for the past 3 weeks. Also called serum fructosamine.

glycemic index. A ranking of carbohydrate-containing foods, based on the food's effect on blood glucose compared with a standard reference food.

glycogen. The form of glucose found in the liver and muscles.

glycosuria. The presence of an abnormal amount of sugar in the urine.

glycosylated hemoglobin. Also known as the A1C, this test measures the average blood glucose level of the past 2 to 3 months.

human chorionic gonadotropin (HCG). A hormone produced by the chorion, which is the membrane enclosing the fetus. It is used shortly after conception, to confirm a pregnancy.

human placental lactogen. A hormone produced by the placenta. The test is used to evaluate how well the placenta is functioning.

hydrocephaly. An abnormal increase in the amount of cerebrospinal fluid within the cranial cavity that is accompanied by expansion of the cerebral ventricles, enlargement of the skull and especially the forehead, and atrophy of the brain.

hyperbilirubinemia. The presence of an excess bilirubin in the blood.

hyperemesis gravidarum. Excessive vomiting during pregnancy.

hyperglycemia. An abnormally high concentration of glucose in the circulating blood.

hyperinsulinemia. The presence of excessive insulin in the blood caused by an overproduction of insulin in the body.

hyperplasia. An abnormal or unusual increase in the elements composing a part.

hypertension. Abnormally high arterial blood pressure.

hypocalcemia. Abnormally low levels of calcium in the circulating blood.

hypoglycemia. An abnormally small concentration of glucose in the circulating blood.

hypomagnesemia. A deficiency of magnesium in the blood.

hypoxia. A deficiency of oxygen in inspired gases or in arterial blood and/or in the tissues.

impaired fasting glucose (IFG). A condition in which a blood glucose test, taken after an 8- to 12-hour fast, shows a level of glucose of 100 mg/dL to 125 mg/dL.

impaired glucose tolerance (IGT). A condition in which blood glucose levels are 140 mg/dL to 199 mg/dL 2 hours after an oral glucose tolerance test (OGTT).

incompetent cervix. Uterine cervix that becomes dilated before term and without labor, frequently resulting in miscarriage or premature birth.

insulin. A protein pancreatic hormone, secreted by the islets of Langerhans, which is essential especially for the metabolism of carbohydrates and is used in the treatment and control of diabetes mellitus.

insulin analog. A tailored form of insulin in which certain amino acids in the insulin molecule have been modified.

insulin pen. An insulin-injecting device that looks like a fountain pen and holds replaceable cartridges of insulin.

insulin pump. An insulin-delivering device, about the size of a deck of cards, which can be worn on a belt or kept in a pocket. It connects to narrow, flexible, plastic tubing (cannula) that ends with a needle inserted just under the skin.

insulin resistance. The body's inability to respond to and use the insulin it produces. Insulin resistance may be linked to obesity, hypertension, and high levels of fat in the blood.

insulin sensitivity. An increase in the effect of the hormone insulin or muscle and adipose tissues.

intrauterine growth retardation (IUGR). Occurs when the fetus is at or below the 10th percentile for weight forage (in weeks).

ketoacidosis. Acidosis caused by the enhanced production of ketone bodies.

ketonemia. A condition marked by an abnormal increase of ketone bodies in the circulating blood.

ketones. An organic compound (such as acetone) with a carbonyl group attached to two carbon atoms.

ketonuria. A condition occurring when ketones are present in the urine, which is a warning sign of diabetic ketoacidosis.

ketosis. An abnormal increase of ketone bodies in conditions of reduced or disturbed carbohydrate metabolism, as in uncontrolled diabetes mellitus.

lancet. A spring-loaded device used to prick the skin with a small needle, to obtain a drop of blood for blood glucose monitoring.

lente insulin. An intermediate-acting insulin that starts to lower blood glucose levels within 1 to 2 hours after injection. It has its strongest effect 8 to 12 hours after injection but keeps working for 18 to 24 hours after injection.

lipid profile. Blood test that measures total cholesterol, triglycerides, and HDL cholesterol.

lipoatrophy. An allergic reaction to insulin medication that is manifested as a loss of subcutaneous fat.

lipohypertrophy. Buildup of fat below the surface of the skin, causing lumps. Lipohypertrophy may be caused by repeated injections of insulin in the same spot.

lispro insulin. See *rapid-acting insulin.*

macrosomia. Refers to abnormally large babies whose mothers may have diabetes.

mannitol. A slightly sweet crystalline alcohol, $C_6H_{14}O_6$, found in many plants and used especially as a diuretic and in testing kidney function.

maternal serum alpha fetal protein. *See* alpha fetoprotein.

metabolic syndrome. Also known as syndrome X, it is the tendency of several conditions, including obesity, insulin resistance, diabetes or prediabetes, hypertension, and high lipids, to occur together.

metformin. An oral medicine used to treat type 2 diabetes. It lowers blood glucose by reducing the amount of glucose the liver produces and by helping the body respond better to the insulin made in the pancreas. Belongs to the class of medicines called biguanides.

nephropathy. An abnormal state of the kidney.

nifedipine. A calcium channel blocker, $C_{17}H_{18}N_2O_6$, that is a coronary vasodilator, used especially in the treatment of angina pectoris.

nonstress test. A test of fetal well-being that is performed by ultrasound monitoring of the increase in fetal heartbeat after fetal movement.

normoglycemia. The presence of a normal concentration of glucose in the blood.

NPH insulin (neutral protamine Hagedorn). An intermediate-acting insulin that starts to lower blood glucose within 1 to 2 hours after injection. It has its strongest effect 6 to 10 hours after injection but keeps working about 18 hours after injection.

oligohydramnios. A deficiency of amniotic fluid sometimes resulting in embryonic defect through adherence between embryo and amnion.

oral glucose tolerance test (OGTT). A test to diagnose prediabetes and diabetes. The oral glucose tolerance test is given after an overnight fast. A fasting blood sample is taken, then the patient drinks a high-glucose beverage. Blood samples are taken at various intervals for 2 to 3 hours. Test results are compared with a standard and show how the body uses glucose over time.

perinatal. Occurring in or concerned with the period around the time of birth.

placenta previa. An abnormal implantation of the placenta at or near the internal opening of the uterine cervix, which tends to precede the child at birth, usually causing severe maternal hemorrhage.

polycystic ovary disease. A condition characterized by enlarged ovaries with multiple small cysts, an abnormally high number of follicles at various states of maturation, and a thick, scarred capsule surrounding each ovary.

polycythemia. A condition marked by an abnormal increase in the number of circulating red blood cells.

polydipsia. Excessive thirst.

polyhydramnios. Excessive accumulation of the amniotic fluid.

polyuria. Excessive urination.

postprandial. Occurring after a meal.

prediabetes. A condition in which blood glucose levels are higher than normal but are not high enough for a diagnosis of diabetes.

preeclampsia. A toxic condition developing in late pregnancy, characterized by a sudden rise in blood pressure, excessive weight gain, generalized edema, albuminuria, severe headache, and visual disturbances.

premature rupture of membranes (PROM). An event that occurs during pregnancy, when the sac containing the developing baby (fetus) and the amniotic fluid bursts or develops a hole before the start of labor.

preprandial. Preceding a meal.

preterm labor. Onset of labor with effacement and dilation of the cervix before the 37th week of gestation.

prolactin. A protein hormone of the anterior lobe of the pituitary gland that induces lactation and maintains the corpora lutea in a functioning state.

prostaglandin synthesis inhibitors. *See* tocolysis agent.

rapid-acting insulin. Insulin that starts to lower blood glucose within 5 to 10 minutes after injection and has its strongest effect 30 minutes to 3 hours after injection, depending on the type used.

regular insulin. *See* short-acting insulin.

respiratory distress syndrome. A respiratory disease of unknown cause that occurs in newborn premature infants and is characterized by deficiency of the surfactant coating the inner surface of the lungs, by failure of the lungs to expand and contract properly during breathing with resulting collapse, and by the accumulation of a protein-containing film lining the alveoli and their ducts.

saccharin. A crystalline imide, $C_7H_5NO_3S$, that is unrelated to carbohydrates, is several hundred times sweeter than cane sugar, and is used as an energy-free sweetener.

serum fructosamine. *See* glycated serum protein.

short-acting insulin. A type of insulin that starts to lower blood glucose within 30 minutes after injection and has its strongest effect 2 to 5 hours after injection.

sorbitol. A faintly sweet alcohol, $C_6H_{14}O_6$, which occurs especially in fruits of the mountain ash, is made synthetically, and is used especially as a humectant, a softener and a sweetener, and in making ascorbic acid.

stevia. A sugar substitute originating from the stevia plant.

sucralose. A sweetener made from sugar but with no calories and no nutritional value.

sugar alcohols. Sweeteners that produce a smaller rise in blood glucose than other carbohydrates.

sulfonylurea. A class of oral medicine for type 2 diabetes that lowers blood glucose by helping the pancreas make more insulin and by helping the body to better use the insulin it makes.

teratogenic. Relating to or causing developmental malformations.

thiazolidinedione. A class of oral medication for type 2 diabetes that helps insulin take glucose from the blood into the cells for energy by making cells more sensitive to insulin.

tocolytics. Any drug treatment modality designed to inhibit uterine contractions in pregnant women at risk for preterm labor.

ultralente insulin. A long-acting insulin that starts to lower blood glucose within 4 to 6 hours after injection. Its strongest effect is 10 to 18 hours after injection, and it keeps working 24 to 28 hours after injection.

ultrasonography. The diagnostic or therapeutic use of ultrasound and especially a technique involving the formation of a two-dimensional image used for the examination and measurement of internal body structures and the detection of bodily abnormalities.

very-long-acting insulin. Insulin that starts to lower blood glucose within 1 hour after injection and keeps working evenly for 24 hours after injection.

xylitol. Carbohydrate-based sweetener found in plants and used as a substitute for sugar; provides calories.

INDEX

Page numbers with *b* indicate boxes; with *f,* figures; and with *t,* tables.